Lifestyle Performance

A Model for Engaging the
Power of Occupation

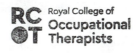
Lifestyle Performance

A Model for Engaging the
Power of Occupation

Beth P. Velde, PhD, OTR/L

East Carolina University
Greenville, North Carolina

Gail S. Fidler, OTR, FAOTA

Pompano Beach, Florida

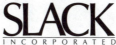

SLACK
INCORPORATED

an innovative information, education, and management company

6900 Grove Road • Thorofare, NJ 08086

The procedures and practices described in this book should be implemented in a manner consistent with the professional standards set for the circumstances that apply in each specific situation. Every effort has been made to confirm the accuracy of the information presented and to correctly relate generally accepted practices. The author, editor, and publisher cannot accept responsibility for errors or exclusions or for the outcome of the application of the material presented herein. There is no expressed or implied warranty of this book or information imparted by it.

The work SLACK publishes is peer reviewed. Prior to publication, recognized leaders in the field, educators, and clinicians provide important feedback on the concepts and content that we publish. We welcome feedback on this work.

Printed in the United States of America
ISBN 1-55642-466-3

Published by: SLACK Incorporated
                 6900 Grove Road
                 Thorofare, NJ 08086 USA
                 Telephone: 856-848-1000
                 Fax: 856-853-5991
                 www.slackbooks.com

Contact SLACK Incorporated for more information about other books in this field or about the availability of our books from distributors outside the United States.

Last digit is print number: 10   9   8   7   6   5   4   3   2   1

ABOUT THE COVER

The painting on the cover is a depiction of artist Sue Hand's interpretation of the Lifestyle Performance Model. Hand, of Sue Hand's Imagery in Dallas, PA, sees the concept of lifestyle as an interactive mosaic of people, environments, and occupations. The four persons in the foreground appear to be purposefully entering a setting filled with individuals who are occupied by a variety of activities, some solitary and some interpersonal.

Each activity holds unique meaning to the performer and it is this creation of meaning that determines the Lifestyle Performance domain in which that activity best fits. Hand has painted the physical environment to include natural and man-made settings. The path flows forward as the four enter the scene. Yet, she has included a section of the path behind them portraying the temporal link inherent in a lifestyle. The social and cultural aspects of the environment are portrayed by the variety of people and objects in the painting.

The potential that the model has for intervention purposes and for wellness is presented subtly by drawing the viewer to closely examine the artist's subjects. Are there persons in the painting who have disabilities? Is the artist suggesting that when viewing lifestyle through the Lifestyle Performance Model a person's strengths are clearly visible and deficits difficult to see as the environments and occupations join to create a supportive and individualistic lifestyle?

DEDICATION

To my family for their support, understanding, and personification of
what human engagement in occupation truly means.
Beth P. Velde

To my daughter, Dagny, and my son, Eric, who give to me everlasting joy,
pride, and love and who personify the quality in living.
Gail S. Fidler

CONTENTS

The *Lifestyle Performance Instructor's Manual* is also available from SLACK Incorporated. Don't miss this important companion to *Lifestyle Performance: A Model for Engaging the Power of Occupation.* To obtain the instructor's manual, please visit http://www.efacultylounge.com.

ACKNOWLEDGMENTS

This book could not have been completed without the editorial assistance of Sharon Elliott, Lara Lancaster, and Dr. Sherrilene Classen, nor would it have ever made it to press without the patience and understanding of the professionals at SLACK Incorporated. Our co-authors in Chapters 9 through 15 provide our readers with real life examples of the model at work. Our thanks to all!

ABOUT THE AUTHORS

Beth P. Velde, PhD, OTR/L is director of graduate studies and associate professor of occupational therapy at East Carolina University, Greenville, NC. Dr. Velde earned a bachelor of science degree in zoology and a master of science degree in parks and recreation from the University of Illinois, a master of science degree in occupational therapy from College Misericordia, Dallas, PA, and a PhD in educational psychology from the University of Calgary, Alberta. Since becoming an occupational therapist, she has authored 25 scholarly papers, chapters, and books, including *Activities: Reality and Symbol* and *Community Occupational Therapy Education and Practice.* Her special interest is in community-built occupational therapy practice and research into the relationship of occupation in quality of life.

Gail S. Fidler, OTR, FAOTA holds a bachelor of arts degree from Lebanon Valley College, Annville, PA, and received her formal education in occupational therapy at the University of Pennsylvania. Her early years as an occupational therapist were spent at military and veteran's hospitals. She has worked for the American Occupational Therapy Association as coordinator of the Psychiatric Study Group and has held numerous positions with occupational therapy educational programs. Mrs. Fidler has published over 25 articles and chapters, and has authored or co-authored six books, including *Activities: Reality and Symbol.* She continues to pursue scholarly activities in occupational therapy and present her ideas through a variety of modalities.

CONTRIBUTING AUTHORS

Michael Amory, MS, OTR/L
Department of Physical Medicine & Rehabilitation
St. Luke's Hospital
Bethlehem, PA

Peter Balent, OTR/L
Lenoir Memorial Hospital
Kinston, NC

Amy Flowers, OTR/L
Pitt County Schools
Greenville, NC

Amy Gerney, MS, OTR/L
Hughesville, PA

Matt Stinson, OTR/L
Caswell Center, OT Department
Kinston, NC

Peggy P. Wittman, EdD, OTR/L, FAOTA
Department of Occupational Therapy
East Carolina University
Greenville, NC

INTRODUCTION

Why Use the Lifestyle Performance Model?

As an occupational therapy student, I was placed in a nursing home setting where we had no clinic space and limited equipment and materials. Most of our care was done in hallways, residents' rooms, and the day room. Whenever we could, we took residents into the courtyard or on short trips into the city. I was particularly struck by Kathleen, an 85-year-old widow. Prior to being admitted to this facility, she had spent 10 years in a state psychiatric facility. Earlier in her life she was a parent and wife. Her son lived in the same state within a 3-hour drive of the nursing home. Her granddaughter lived approximately 5 hours away. She had grandchildren, although the number and sex are unclear from her records.

Kathleen shared a room with two other female residents. She had several pictures of her family on her nightstand drawer. Her clothing was stored in two drawers in a shared dresser and in a locker located in the room. Her room had a grooming area with a sink and bathroom with toilet and bathtub. She had no other personal objects in her room. Staff and residents alike complained of Kathleen's pinching and hitting behaviors. Most people believed she was both non-verbal and mentally handicapped.

Many occupational therapy strategies had been attempted with Kathleen with minimal success. I hoped that by using the Lifestyle Performance Model, I could both reach Kathleen and demonstrate to staff and other residents her value as a human being. My goal was to enhance her quality of life by using the constructs and sub-constructs of the Lifestyle Performance Model. This is Kathleen's abbreviated occupational story.

Self-Care and Self-Maintenance

Prior to beginning occupational therapy treatment, Kathleen was dependent on staff for all personal grooming, bathing, and dressing. She was in a standard wheelchair with a Velcro seatbelt, footrests, and wedge cushion. Her posture was poor, slouching in the chair with a posterior pelvic tilt. She spent much of her day in bed due to skin breakdown on her legs and buttocks. She moved her wheelchair only short distances using her arms. Moving from sit to stand required a two-person maximum assistance. She was able to stand for less than 10 seconds.

Kathleen fed herself and drank independently. She ate in the main dining room of the residence, sitting with three to four other residents. She did not have teeth or dentures and consequently ate puréed foods. Her medications were managed by the charge nurse. She took them willingly. At the time of the occupational therapy assessment, Kathleen was taking resperidal, tamoxifen, Synthroid, multivitamins, procardin, neutraphospate, Depakote, Paxil, and Haldol.

She had resperidal prescribed on an as-needed basis. Her diagnoses included hypertension, hypothyroidism, non-insulin-dependent diabetes, seizure disorder, cataracts, deafness, neurogenic bladder, post-fracture of the right humerus, schizophrenia, and depression.

It was important to me to increase her autonomy in the area of self-care/self-maintenance. After using occupational therapy strategies of remediation (strengthening, postural), compensation (adapting equipment and materials), and education (of Kathleen and staff), her autonomy improved. For example, when given the opportunity by the nursing staff, she chose her own clothing and assisted with upper extremity dressing. She enjoyed combing her hair and washing with set-up and minimal assistance. With set-up and moderate assistance, she applied nail polish. Kathleen moved to a wheelchair without footrests and propelled herself throughout the facility using her arms and feet. She was able to reposition herself in her chair when cued, and reports of skin breakdown were reduced. She maintained an upright, seated posture. She was able to move from sit to stand with moderate assistance and monitoring for safety, and stood with support for 1 minute. She walked with restorative nursing staff using a rolling walker and two-person assistance.

Societal Contribution

Prior to being admitted to the state psychiatric facility, Kathleen was a housewife. Since her admittance to long-term care, she has not worked or volunteered. According to her records and to current nursing staff, she did not assist with her care or the care of her possessions.

After working with volunteers and staff regarding her needs in this domain, staff better understood why it was important to take the time to allow Kathleen to participate in nursing home life. Staff began to ask Kathleen for "help" with a task. While these requests were simple ones, such as "help us stand you up," she smiled when she could comply. She frequently stated, "I helped you," after completing a task.

Intrinsic Gratification

Kathleen spent most of her time in bed or sitting in her wheelchair in the hallway. She did not attend activity programs. Staff reported she seldom smiled. I began working with the activity staff and attending appropriate activity groups with Kathleen. She was able to do simple crafts with cues and participate as an observer in games. Volunteers were secured and trained in assisting her so she could maintain her participation in the activity program. In addition, I began working with Kathleen using acrylic paints and canvas as a way for her to express herself. She kept these works of art on display in her room—the only objects of a personal nature that were visible.

Reciprocal Interpersonal Relatedness

There were pictures of her family in the drawer of her bedside table, yet she indicated she did not know who they were. She received cards at "family-based" holidays. When seated in the hall, she reached out and grabbed staff and other residents as they went by. She shared a room with two women, one of whom was verbal and had potential for interaction with Kathleen. Since moving to the facility, Kathleen demonstrated no spontaneous verbal communication. Her receptive communication was excellent when the speaker attended to her hearing problem.

It was important to me that Kathleen develop more positive ways of getting attention and interaction with staff and other residents. Part of this was achieved with the activity program. In addition, I began providing services to one of her roommates and intervention sessions included both women. We worked on a variety of activities that required what Moore and Anderson called games of strategy (e.g., simple gross motor games and some table games). I also asked the nursing staff to add her to the residents looking for an adoption—a volunteer or staff member who would spend extra time with her and provide her with simple gifts at appropriate times. Staff reported that her incidents of hitting and pinching decreased.

Outcomes

My interaction with Kathleen was a positive experience. As a novice occupational therapist, it demonstrated to me the power of occupation and the need to find a way to practice that was holistically oriented. I discovered that the Lifestyle Performance Model allowed me to treat people as typical—viewing their strengths and addressing their needs when they interfered with the person's quality of life. The model made me address Kathleen's environment and taught me that "fixing the person" was a very limited way to practice occupational therapy.

The intent of this book is to empower therapists to use the model and to learn new ways of being client-centered. It is not intended to suggest that the way therapists are practicing is wrong, but to investigate whether there might be a better way!

—Beth P. Velde, PhD, OTR/L

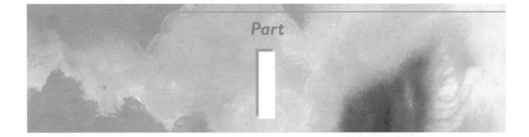

OVERVIEW OF THE
LIFESTYLE PERFORMANCE MODEL

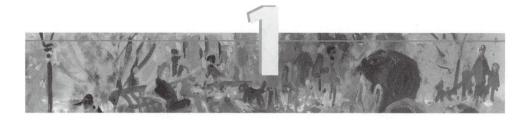

Understanding the Lifestyle Performance Model in the Occupational Therapy Context

The Lifestyle Performance Model contends that users of the model can engage the power of occupation to enhance quality of life. But what is the power of occupation? Paul, a young adult with quadriplegia, describes his perception of occupation's power as

> going into another state of thinking. And, you know, I find a form of euphoria after… I think what you can produce under those circumstances goes far beyond what you can in a forced situation because the romance is there, you know, your heart is into it, your mind is into it, your total being is into what you're doing.

Using tenets of the Lifestyle Performance Model, the power of occupation—of achieving the state described by Paul—occurs when there is congruence between the characteristics of an individual and the characteristics of an activity.

Why should occupational therapists use occupation's power in practice? Occupation's power is unleashed when the requirements of an activity approximate a person's neurobiology, psychological structure, and skills, and meets the individual's needs. Persons are not always able to choose activities that address these criteria. This may occur because of an existing health condition or acquired impairment, a lack of self-knowledge, a failure of the environment to support engagement in activity, or a mismatch between the demands of the environment on an individual and his or her activity skills. What is the outcome of using the power of occupation in practice? Perhaps the most desired effect is an enhanced quality of life.

STRUCTURE OF THE TEXT

This text describes the varying dimensions of the Lifestyle Performance Model in an effort to enable graduate students, practitioners, and faculty to gain an understanding that will support the application of the model and its further research. The Lifestyle Performance Model has evolved over more than three decades of study, trial, and reassessment.

The text is divided into two parts: The first section is concerned with explaining the fundamental theoretical construct of the model—its form, structure, and rationale. This is followed by an explanation of the components of the model. The second section of the text presents examples of application of the model, spanning a variety of settings; each is presented by the occupational therapist engaged in the intervention. The book concludes by addressing the need for further research.

HOW DOES THE MODEL DIFFER FROM OTHER OCCUPATIONAL THERAPY MODELS?

Persons approach a new learning opportunity with a set of assumptions and expectations. These assumptions and expectations relate to their prior learning concerning the stated subject matter. Thus, it is reasonable to expect that a learning experience designed to explain the rationale and processes of the Lifestyle Performance Model will follow this premise. Therefore, it is critical to begin this learning experience with an awareness that the Lifestyle Performance Model differs from other occupational therapy models of practice in terms of both focus and process.

The model's underlying philosophy and belief system profess that the quality of life is the single most important focus in living; identification, support, and development of an individual's strengths, skills, and interests enhance the quality of that life. Therefore, the first and most significant concern of the model is to identify a person's performed strengths, capacity, and interests, and to collaboratively plan a daily living repertoire that will use and enhance personal strengths and interests. Performance deficits are secondary concerns addressed only when it can be demonstrated that such limitations significantly interfere with or preclude the pursuit of personal satisfaction and quality of life. When that is determined, then the traditional intervention of relevant remediation and compensation should occur. The Lifestyle Performance Model does not specify a technique or frame of reference for such interventions. The therapist makes the choice of method. Such intervention strategies, however, should not preempt the primary focus and process of the model. The principle concern is what is right about the person, not what is wrong.

Activities are understood and used as total entities, each with their own separate characteristics, sociological meanings, and cultural meanings irrespective of the performer. A given unit or part of an activity is considered a task within the activity, not the activity itself. Activities are acknowledged as having real and symbolic meaning. Activities of daily living encompass those activities that comprise the daily living engagement of an individual. The significant and primary role of activities in the formation and application of the model requires a solid foundation concerning the critical role of activities in the reflection and shaping of cultures and persons. Study of the text *Activities: Reality and Symbol* (Fidler & Velde, 1999) and other similar works should be considered an essential prerequisite to the study and application of the Lifestyle Performance Model.

An activity encompasses a number of elements that contribute to defining the nature and characteristics of the activity. These include form and structure, action processes, properties, discernable outcome, and real and symbolic meaning. To understand the model, it is important to distinguish activity from occupation. While occupation is defined and understood as the dynamic, complex process of being engaged in "doing," it is not a synonym for activity; rather, it connotes the dynamic process of doing. It is the phenomenon of mind and body being occupied.

The environment is an integral part of the structure and operation of the model. The environmental context in which daily living activities occur (e.g., the home, school, workplace, nursing home; the season of the year or time of day; the social group, etc.) are essential dimensions of the model. Data-gathering processes and evaluations include consideration of a given environment's ability to be responsive to human needs and interests.

One of the distinguishing features of the Lifestyle Performance Model is its phenomenological approach. The data-gathering processes rely on observation and interview with the client and, as appropriate, significant others who share or have shared in the client's living experiences. The interview is an open-ended dialogue focused on facilitating the client telling the story of his or her daily living activities. Data gathering regarding a person's daily activity repertoire also includes collaboration with other professionals to access their expertise and perceptions about the individual.

There are no standards of right or wrong, of normal-not normal, no statistical or other measures against which to compare the data. Evaluations are based on an emic perspective. In maintaining this perspective, the practitioner attempts to understand the individual's perspective of reality. This emphasizes the person's capacities, interests, and needs.

This text intends to describe how to engage the power of occupation, describe when and how to use this power, and provide ways to determine if the outcome of its use is truly a lifestyle that is more satisfying than not to self and significant others.

KEY POINTS

- The model works to identify and work with a person's strengths, capacity, and interests, and to collaboratively plan a daily living repertoire to enhance those.
- Occupation is the dynamic process of being engaged in doing an activity.
- Activities have a form and structure, action processes, properties, outcomes, and real and symbolic meaning.
- The model is based in a phenomenological approach.

REFERENCE

Fidler, G. S., & Velde, B. P. (1999). *Activities: Reality and symbol.* Thorofare, NJ: SLACK Incorporated.

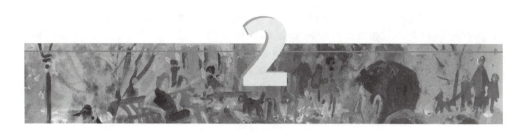

Structure of the Lifestyle Performance Model

The Lifestyle Performance Model is a conceptual framework for the study and the use of activity in the daily lives of individuals, in their institutions, and in society. As such, the model provides a format for discovering the meanings and roles of activities in contributing to quality of life; in shaping human performance and lifestyles; cultivating and mirroring group, community, and societal development; and in formulating and reflecting organization and institutional structure and behaviors.

The model is grounded in those tenets that affirm the power of occupation in human existence. The term *occupation* is used to refer to the process of being occupied, being engaged in a doing experience. It connotes the dynamics of action-focused engagement. This engagement is viewed as the occupational process and understood as a complex dynamic encompassing neurological, psychological, cognitive, and sociocultural phenomena. Csikszentmihalyi (1997) discusses the potential outcome of this engagement as *flow*.

The activities inherent to such processes are acknowledged as total entities having meaning in and of themselves. Each carries a symbolic message as well as a reality-based one. Each is a complex mix of anthropological, historical, physical, psychological, sociocultural, political, and economic variables (Fidler & Velde, 1999). Pierce (2001) suggests a similar distinction between activities and occupation, identifying *activity* as the universally recognized phenomenon and *occupation* as the individualized, contextually bound engagement in activity.

Understanding the significance of the occupational process requires a knowing appreciation of the complex dynamics of activities and their impact on individual and sociocultural development, as well as on organizational structure and operations. Developing this knowledge base is essential for understanding the nature and relevant determinants of a lifestyle that can be expected to contribute to well-being and to quality of life.

MOTIVATION

Certainly one important variant in this process is the role of motivation. Motivation is an internal phenomenon and leads to human behavior. Theories relating to the varied meanings of activities strongly suggest that motivation is triggered and sustained when there is congruence between the characteristics of an individual and the characteristics of an activity. Furthermore, it has been proposed that a sense of mastery and competence is more readily achieved and the sense of intrinsic gratification intensifies when one is engaged with activities whose requirements most closely match one's neurobiology, psychological structure, and skills (Moneta & Csikszentmihalyi, 1996; Fidler, 1981).

The action focus of human behavior is understood as an innate drive to act, explore, and cope with the challenges of one's environment. This drive is essential not only as a means of species survival but particularly as enabling personal and social development. Becoming part of human society involves activity that transforms primitive actions into behaviors that serve personal needs and contribute to the development of society (Fidler & Fidler, 1978; Moore & Anderson, 1968). Validation of one's humanness is a life-long pursuit, and engagement in activities that are personally and socially relevant offers critical on-going verification. A perception of one's personal competence and self-agency (the capacity to change behavior and improve self [Karoly, 1993; Mischel, Cantor, & Feldman, 1996]) derives in good measure from coping with and managing the performance imperatives inherent in activities (similar to the performance mastery discussed by Bandura in 1977). These learning experiences are reinforced and verified in the end product, which provides evidence of achievement.

LIFESTYLE

A personal way of living (e.g., a lifestyle) comprises engagement in a repertoire of daily life activities congruent with individual needs and to the sociocultural norms of that person's society.

> *Each individual, over time, develops a configuration of activity patterns that can be described as a lifestyle. These patterns of doing, of being engaged, emerge through the interplay of a person's intrinsic needs, desires, and capacities, and unique expectations of the environmental context of the person's living. (Fidler, 1996, p. 140)*

Such engagements are intrinsically interwoven with an ever-evolving sense of self and of one's societal membership. The perception of personal competence and self-worth then develops in good measure from coping with and managing the performance imperatives of activities. When such occupational processes include collaboration with others and when performance, for example, is a shared group experience, social role learning and interpersonal skill development are nurtured.

Society exerts a strong influence on how activities are perceived. The status and societal merit of an activity varies in accordance with social values and established norms. Thus, engagement and competency in those activities that are valued by a given society have significant impact on defining personal and social efficacy and tend to be weighted over activities with less status (Fidler, 1981).

WELL-BEING AND QUALITY OF LIFE

An overall sense of satisfaction and a feeling of well-being derives from the sum of the positive benefits gleaned from a daily living activity configuration that is in harmony with self and with those who share in the living experiences. Satisfaction is defined as one's cognitive appraisal of one's lifestyle. It is impacted by one's values and culture. For example, Western culture tends to be individualistic and gives priority to the goals of individuals who feel personally responsible for their successes and failures, and experience some separation and distance from their in-groups (Triandis, McCusker, & Hui, 1990). Well-being is an affective response to the sense of satisfaction. These are related to quality of life.

Quality of life is a phrase replete with subjective, personally unique meanings. Generally speaking, the quality of one's life can be judged by the nature and quality of one's lifestyle (Fidler & Fidler, 1978; 1983). A succinct, unambiguous definition of the term is elusive at best (Raphael, 1997). Current literature, however, does reflect a number of efforts to identify and describe the more salient factors that seem to influence judgment about the quality of one's life.

Hultsman (1985) attributes quality of life to "the amount of perceived freedom, the proportion of motivation which was intrinsic rather than extrinsic, and the amount of positive affect which subjects attributed to various types of life experiences" (p. 5). Brown's (1988) framework incorporates three areas: "The first would pertain to an individual's perception of self; the second to the individual's behaviour in response to ecological domains that might affect him/her; and the third to responses the settings might make to the individual" (p. 174).

Brown, Bayer, and MacFarlane (1989) identify the role of the individual in trying to define quality of life. "Quality of life is an interaction between the individual and the environment. It can be described in terms of personal control that can be exerted by the individual over the environment. It must be assessed by consulting the individual directly" (p. 57). This orientation recognizes the importance of person-environment interactions within a cultural and ecological perspective and supports the contribution of personally relevant activities to quality of life.

Many are now recognizing that quality of life is not equal to functional competence. McKenna (1993) incorporates the need to view quality of life in both generalized terms and as an idiosyncratic interpretation:

> ...I feel that quality of life has some commonalities and can be generalized, but only to a certain extent. Having autonomy and freedom; enjoying self-integrity and self-esteem; being free of illness, pain, or physical restriction are features which would undoubtedly be prized by most people and would almost universally be identified as components of life's goodness. (p. 34)

However, aside from these common denominators, there are those features that are valued to a special degree by the individual alone. To play, to golf, to travel, to hold a grandchild, to feel a oneness with the environment are very personal experiences identified by some participants as being the key to their happiness and quality of life.

A global model represents quality of life using both objective and subjective measures. *Objective criteria* include descriptions of the person's physical environment, social environment, health status, economic stability, and activity configuration. *Subjective criteria* illustrate the individual's perceptions of each objective criterion. This includes feelings about the extent to which his or her needs are being met relative to each objective criteria as well as an overall perception of life satisfaction. Many authors (Felce & Perry, 1997; Brown, Bayer, & MacFarlane, 1989; Quality of Life Research Project, 2000; Zhan, 1992) support a combined model in which both objective and subjective assessments are incorporated. In contrast to models focusing on health and impairment (e.g., Health Related Quality of Life [HRQOL]), a global model addresses quality of life from a wellness perspective. Further, the objective criteria are observable through the activities in which an individual is engaged.

Using such a model, the interpretation of one's quality of life includes:

- ❦ The discrepancy between a person's achieved and unmet needs and desires. These needs and desires are met through the occupational dynamic.

- ❦ The extent to which an individual experiences freedom and control in the activities representing his or her lifestyle.

- ❦ The discrepancy between the lifestyle of the individual and the norms of one's culture regarding an activity.

The congruence between the subjective and objective measures must be considered. For example, if an individual reports a high level of satisfaction with his or her perception of the objective measures—yet the objective measures demonstrate a low achievement in relationship to the norm—this account of quality of life would require further investigation.

CONSTRUCTS OF THE MODEL

The configuration of the Lifestyle Performance Model makes it possible to identify the relationship of activity patterns to the pursuit of a person's unique needs to achieve a personal identity, to understand the activities within the context of the sociocultural norm, and take into account aspects of freedom and control within a person's lifestyle. It provides a focus for study and practice of occupational therapy as a multi-faceted process of enabling a way of living that is intrinsically gratifying as well as socially contributory. The model extends the parameters of occupational therapy beyond reducing disability, beyond the realm of our traditional activities of daily living (ADLs) (Fidler, 1996).

Since the model is concerned with identifying and describing a contextual configuration of daily living activities that will potentially optimize individual wellness and quality of life, its framework comprises two major constructs. The model first considers the activity elements of an environment that can be expected to foster and support the achievement of a satisfying and productive lifestyle. Then, it provides a format for considering the nature and interrelationships of activities that are relevant to the needs and concerns of daily living. It offers a structural perspective for defining a lifestyle in harmony with personal and societal needs and expectations.

THE ENVIRONMENT

The significance of the interplay between person and environment has been well documented in the literature of behavioral and medical sciences. The Lifestyle Performance Model identifies and describes those elements that create a clarifying and responsive environment that supports and facilitates satisfying human endeavors. Within the context of the model, the environment is considered responsive (answers to individual needs and interests), and clarifying (makes reality and expectations knowable) to the extent that its structural and operational activity incorporates and supports opportunities for the following (Fidler, 1996, p. 143):

- Autonomy: to be self-determining, gain a sense of being more in control over one's life than not, to be as self-dependent as personal needs and capacities define.

- Individuality: to be self-differentiating, see and know one's uniqueness; verify the identity of self and confirm the entitlement of one's interests, skills, and differences.

- Affiliation: have evidence of belonging; being part of a group, a dyad, a community; and to know interdependence.

- Volition: to have alternatives, to have access to sufficient information and latitude to make and act on one's choice.

- ❦ Consensual validation: to have feedback on one's actions from others that verify one's perceptions and reality; to be part of reciprocal exchanges that clarify and acknowledge one's contributions and actions.

- ❦ Predictability: to discern and evaluate cause and effect, be able to predict and limit ambiguity and risk, give order to one's world, and experience the comfort of predictability.

- ❦ Self-efficacy: to believe one is able to cope and manage one's everyday living tasks, of being a cause and making things happen.

- ❦ Adventure: to be able to seek and try out the new, the unknown; to explore, look beyond the here and now; and to discover, experiment, dare to risk, be free of the fear of failure.

- ❦ Accommodation: to be free from physical and mental harm; to function in an environment that is responsive to individual capabilities while compensating for individual limitations.

- ❦ Reflections: to have respite from activity, time out to ponder on the meaning of things, to renew the self, and contemplate recent and past events.

These guidelines form the basis for identifying and describing (within the context of a given setting and its purpose) those activities that most readily relate to and support such fundamental needs and that are simultaneously relevant to and facilitate the mission and objectives of the environmental setting. Activity configurations can then be developed for environments such as the home, school, workplace, and health care organization. (The environmental focus of the model is more fully explored in Chapter 5.)

THE FOUR DOMAINS

The second major construct of the model addresses those patterns of occupations that may be said to comprise a way of living that maximizes wellness and quality of living. A lifestyle that is potentially satisfying and socially productive is conceptualized as comprising four occupational domains. It is proposed that these domains represent the principle motives around which daily living is constructed. Each domain is seen as being characterized by activities that are relevant to the focus of the domain, to the unique capacities and interests of the individual, and to social norms.

The four occupational domains encompass:

- ❦ Self-care and self-maintenance: patterns of activities concerned with caring for and maintaining the self in as self-dependent a manner as personal needs and capacities determine.

- ❦ Intrinsic gratification: those activity patterns focused on the pursuit of personal pleasure and enjoyment.

- ❦ Societal contribution: activity patterns concerned with contributing to need fulfillment and the welfare of others.

❦ Reciprocal interpersonal relatedness: those activities focused on developing and sustaining relationships with others.

Fidler (1996) has explained that since "these domains represent the principle focus of daily living activities, they are relevant throughout the life span. What may be described for any one person at any point in time as an adequately balanced lifestyle depends upon the age, culture, and neurobiological endowment of the person as well as the values and resources of the person's social matrix" (p. 144). Lifestyle expectations and interests change with different stages in life and vary in accordance with cultural and social norms. Fidler (1996) furthermore reminds us that although each domain has a distinct focus, they are not independent entities, rather interrelated aspects of daily life. (Exploration of each domain is more fully explored in Chapter 4.)

THE NATURE OF INDIVIDUALIZATION

Certainly there are cultural differences that are manifested in the values assigned to any activity and, therefore, in assigned priorities. Differences are further evident many times in the subtle difference in performance requirements and in the existence of culturally specific activities. For example, rules of games may differ according to locale. The foods and special rituals of universal holidays may vary in different regions of the same country. Age-related variances in the characteristics and performance imperatives as well as choices of activities among age-related populations are most often self-evident. Regardless of these variables, there is ample documentation attesting to the indigenous and essential role of activities in all cultures and throughout civilization.

It is critical to understand that the ways in which the characteristics of an activity are experienced and the reasons for a person's engagement are highly individualized dynamics. Activities cannot be categorized as belonging to any one domain. In a uniquely human manner, persons select activities based on what the activity characteristics mean to them in terms of their needs and interests and the sociocultural norms of their society.

THE NATURE OF INTERVENTION

Within the conceptual framework of the model, evaluation and assessment are predominantly a phenomenological process. Information that must form the basis of any plan or application is best gathered from personal interviews. Whether the model is applied as a wellness-enhancing or remedial intervention, the first concern is to define and describe the person's customary lifestyle activity patterns. Interventions and outcome expectations are formulated on the basis of the person's strengths, skills, interests, and resources, and the expectations of significant others. A fundamental concept of the model is that dysfunction and any treatment initiative can be defined only from the perspective of what constitutes a person's quality of life. Dysfunction is an individually referenced state of being, defined at any one point in time by personal, social, and cultural variables.

Strengths and limitations in sensory processing, motor function, cognition, psychological structure, and interpersonal perceptions are certainly important variables in the development and sustainment of activity patterns. When one or more occupational domains of a person's lifestyle are affected by trauma to these systems, remedial intervention is, of course, necessary; and traditional evaluation processes are in order. However, the Lifestyle Performance Model extends occupational therapy intervention beyond addressing an impairment. Its principle focus is to work with the person to develop or redevelop a lifestyle pattern of activities that will enhance the quality of that person's life. In some instances, this endeavor will mean establishing a more satisfying lifestyle. In others, it will involve restoring a previously achieved lifestyle (Fidler, 1996).

Developing an occupational therapy plan to enhance wellness or for prevention or remediation includes (Fidler, 1996, p. 145):

- The development of a Lifestyle Performance Profile reflecting what is or what has been the person's typical lifestyle activity pattern.
- A description of current performance abilities and limitations relative to each.
- The performance expectations and preferences of self and significant others in relationship to each domain.
- The balance and harmony among the domains within the context of age, and social and cultural norms.
- Family and community sociocultural values, expectations, economic resources, and limitations.
- Evaluation of any performance component that notably affects one or more domains.
- Individual characteristics, interests, values, and abilities that shape performance.
- Design of a recommended Lifestyle Performance Profile that reflects current capacities, needs, and interests.

Understanding the relevance of occupation to human development, to health maintenance and restoration, and to the quality of life is the unending mission of occupational therapy. As Fidler (1996) reminds us, such pursuit involves exploration of the complex mix of anthropological, historical, physical, psychological, sociocultural, economic, and political variables of the person-activity dynamic. The science of occupation must seek to explain how these dynamics of doing, of being occupied, relate to the dimensions of physical integrity, psychological structure, and social relatedness. Our scientific base must furthermore strive to explain how these phenomena generate the ability and drive to fulfill personally relevant activities and roles of everyday living in ways that are mutually satisfying to the self and to those who comprise one's social matrix. The Lifestyle Performance Model offers a framework for the study and testing of such relationships.

KEY POINTS

* The key construct of the model is lifestyle.
* Lifestyle is composed of self-care/self-maintenance, intrinsic gratification, reciprocal interpersonal relatedness, and societal contributions.
* Activities in the four domains can be supported and/or constrained by the environment.
* When the daily living activity configuration is in harmony, then a perception of quality of life follows.
* Evaluation and assessment are essentially a phenomenological process.

REFERENCES

Bandura, A. (1977). Self-efficacy: Toward a unifying theory of behavioral change. *Psychological Review, 84*, 191-215.

Brown, M. (1988). Consequences of impairment on activity. *Rehabilitation Psychology, 33*(2), 173-184.

Brown, R. I., Bayer, M. B., & MacFarlane, C. (1989). *Rehabilitation programmes: Performance and quality of life of adults with developmental handicaps.* Toronto, ON: Lugus Productions Ltd.

Csikszentmihalyi, M. (1997). *Finding flow.* New York: Harper Collins Publishers, Inc.

Felce, D., & Perry, J. (1997). In R. I. Brown (Ed.), *Quality of life for people with disabilities* (2nd Ed., pp. 49-62). London: Stanley Thornes.

Fidler, G. S. (1996). Lifestyle performance: From profile to conceptual model. *Am J Occup Ther, 50,* 139-147.

Fidler, G. S. (1981). From crafts to competence. *Am J Occup Ther, 35,* 567-573.

Fidler, G. S., & Fidler, J. W. (1983). Doing and becoming: The occupational therapy experience. In G. Kielhofner (Ed.), *Health through occupation: Theory and practice in occupational therapy* (pp. 267-280). Philadelphia: F. A. Davis.

Fidler, G. S., & Fidler, J. W. (1978). Doing and becoming: Purposeful action and self-actualization. *Am J Occup Ther, 32,* 305-310.

Fidler, G. S., & Velde, B. P. (1999). *Activities: Reality and symbol.* Thorofare, NJ: SLACK Incorporated.

Hultsman, J. (1985). *The relationship of the study of leisure to the perception of quality of life* [microform]. University of Oregon.

Karoly, P. (1993). Mechanisms of self-regulation: A systems view. *Annu Rev Psychol, 44,* 23-52.

McKenna, K. (1993). Quality of Life: A question of functional outcomes or the fulfillment of life plans. *Australian Occupational Therapy Journal, 40*(1), 33-35.

Mischel, W., Cantor, N., & Feldman, S. (1996). The nature of willpower and self-control. In E. T. Higgins & A. W. Kruglanski (Eds.), *Social psychology: Handbook of basic principles* (pp. 329-360). New York: Guilford.

Moneta, G. B., & Csikszentmihalyi, M. (1996). The effect of perceived challenges and skills on the quality of subjective experience. *Journal of Personality, 64*, 275-311.

Moore, O. K., & Anderson, A. R. (1968). *Some principles for the design of clarifying educational environments.* Pittsburgh, PA: University of Pittsburgh, Learning Research and Development Center.

Pierce, D. (2001). Untangling occupation and activity. *Am J Occup Ther, 55*, 138-146.

Quality of Life Research Project. (2000). Retrieved 11/14/00, from http: www. utoronto.ca/qol.

Raphael, D. (1997). Defining quality of life. Eleven debates concerning its measurement. In R. Renwick, I. Brown, & M. Nagler (Eds.), *Quality of life in health promotion and rehabilitation: Conceptual approaches, issues and applications* (pp. 146-170). Thousand Oaks, CA: Sage.

Triandis, H. C., McCusker, C., & Hui, C. H. (1990). Multimethod probes of individualism and collectivism. *J Pers Soc Psychol, 59*, 1006-1020.

Zhan, L. (1992). Quality of life: Conceptual and measurement issues. *J Adv Nurs, 17*, 795-800.

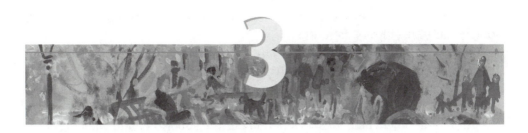

The Model's Relationship to Theory

The Lifestyle Performance Model has evolved over a period of many years (Fidler, 1996; Nelson, 1997), reflecting throughout its development Fidler's steadfast pursuit to understand and articulate the role of activities in the lives of individuals and in shaping and reflecting societies. Harbingers of the model are evident in many of her publications and offer a foundation for understanding this model and its application in practice (Miller & Walker, 1993). The American Occupational Therapy Association's (1997) *Psychosocial Core of Occupational Therapy Position Paper* provides a concise and thorough overview of the essence of the Lifestyle Performance Model.

Theory is the foundation of model building and may be defined as a systematic explanation of an event in which constructs and concepts are identified and relationships are proposed or predictions made (Morse & Field, 1995). Theories are useful because they provide a way to explain reality. Morse and Field suggest that theory provides explanations for what could be seemingly unrelated facts "in the most effective and parsimonious configuration" (1995, p. 5). In other words, a theory can provide clues about what is important, what is superfluous, and what can be set aside regarding the practice of occupational therapy.

Authorities divide theory into grand, mid-range, and low-order theories based on the number of phenomena that the theory is meant to explain (Straus & Corbin, 1990). Texts in occupational therapy use the phrases *model of practice* and *frame of reference.* The phrases are interpreted differently. A comparison of four sources illustrates these differences.

Mosey (1992) describes a model of practice as having three components:

1. Concepts (abstract category delineated by specific characteristics)

2. Definitions (label of the concept, immediate super-ordinate category to which the concept belongs, specific characteristics distinguishing the concept from any other categories included under the super-ordinate category)

3. Postulates (relationships of each concept to others are described: temporal, spatial, quantitative, qualitative, correlative, causal)

A model, according to Mosey, is a broad outline of a profession as understood by both society and the profession. It demonstrates the way in which a profession sees itself in regard to other professions; sees itself in association with society; and describes its philosophical assumptions, ethical code, theoretical foundation, domain(s) of concern, legitimate tools, and nature and sequencing of aspects of practice.

Mosey (1992) describes a frame of reference as an integrated system of postulates that describe an element of the profession's domain of concern, components of that element (if any), and environmental factors that positively influence the element. A frame of reference is a lower level of theory that identifies a specific state of function or dysfunction, including the behavioral and physical signs. It hypothesizes ways of enhancing function and/or modifying dysfunction in the specified area and includes postulates regarding the change.

For Kielhofner (1992; 1995), the appropriate term for the broader collection of assumptions within a profession is *paradigm*. A paradigm is a way to organize and develop knowledge about occupation *per se* using basic and applied research. While it does not provide specifics for practice, it does consist of core assumptions, a focal viewpoint, and the values of the profession. In contrast and at a lower level of theory is what he terms the *conceptual model of practice.* These models "contain(s) theory that serves as the rationale for some aspect of occupational therapy practice" (1995, p. 2). The model has a specific focus and is not intended to serve "all of the multiple factors involved in the occupational functioning of any patient or client" (p. 2).

Miller (1993) suggests a third perspective: the organization of the foundations of knowledge as occurring at various levels. Concepts represent, through symbolic language, phenomena in the environment. These concepts, when related to each other through principles, present an organizational structure that is used to explain and predict. The theory consists not only of sub-concepts, concepts, and principles, it also includes assumptions. The knowledge base of a profession consists of a number of theories.

McColl and Pranger (1994) propose a different description. They distinguish between a conceptual model and a model of practice. "A conceptual model refers to a theoretical tool that helps to explain or predict a central construct, that helps to understand how constructs relate to one another, and promotes an understanding of a central construct" (p. 251). An example of such a construct could be occupation. A model of practice relates to the application of discipline-specific theories to the everyday functioning of a practitioner within a discipline.

For the purpose of this text, the phrase *model of practice* will be used and defined as "a coherent, internally unified way of thinking about... events and processes" (Frank, 1968, p. 45). It is formal theory at a grander level. It is meant to incorporate the body of knowledge or conceptual foundation of occupational therapy at the broadest level. It includes a philosophical stance, concepts, propositions about the relationships between concepts, and a way of organizing the concepts into a structure relevant for occupational therapy. Frames of reference represent lower levels of theory relevant to specific domain(s) of concern.

Theory is developed both inductively and deductively. The inductive process is frequently associated with the positivist paradigm and deduction with the qualitative paradigm.

Morse (1989) describes these differences as follows:

> *Work in the positivist paradigm is usually linear and is seen to proceed logically from previously established knowledge. The starting point is a highly structured view of the phenomenon of interest. The conduct of research serves to verify or refute previous knowledge that was held to be provisional in nature.*

> *...In the qualitative paradigm, the knowing occurs at a different point in the process. In this case the starting point for investigation is typically a somewhat undifferentiated view. The conduct of the research serves to move the analyst to a simultaneously more differentiated and abstract view of the phenomenon (which is the product and may be called "understanding," "rich description," or "theory"). How the scientist comes to this more abstract view is the process as well as the substance of the research. (p. 14)*

The inclusion of research and ways of knowing using many methods and representing more than one research paradigm serves to strengthen theory development in occupational therapy.

THE LIFESTYLE PERFORMANCE MODEL

As a formal theory (Straus & Corbin, 1990), the Lifestyle Performance Model seeks to explain the role of activities in both shaping and reflecting the quality of life of individuals, groups, and organizations within an environmental context. Its concepts include activities or occupations, the occupational process, the dynamics of activities, motivation for behavior, lifestyle, quality of life, the responsive environment, and the four domains of activities. The postulates are based within a phenomenological framework and consist of the relationships between and among the concepts listed above. The concepts and postulates are further described in Chapter 2, *Structure of the Lifestyle Performance Model.*

Its application to an individual represents how a lifestyle is experienced through a repertoire of activities that simultaneously influence the actor and the environment through the engagement in activities. For the actor, engagement in an activity occurs due to one or more reason(s): to achieve intrinsic gratification and pleasure, to contribute to others, to maintain and care for self, or to engage in reciprocal relationships. For any given engagement in an experience, one or more of these reasons may be present in varying degrees.

The model can also be applied to the structure of organizations and the activities inherent in their structure. In this case, the interaction between the environments (physical, social, political, temporal) both support specific activities and are influenced by those activities.

PHENOMENOLOGY AS THE PHILOSOPHICAL STANCE OF THE LIFESTYLE PERFORMANCE MODEL

When engagement in human occupation is viewed as part of the social interaction of human beings (whether specific individuals or organizations of individuals) within a social, political, temporal, and physical context, the meaning may vary based upon the environment. This approach to engagement parallels the assumptions upon which phenomenology is based. These assumptions include the existence of multiple realities, the interrelationship of actor and context, and the difficulty in drawing generalizable *a priori* statements of universal truth.

Phenomenology uses the designation of *life-world*, referring to the world as lived by the person. The life-world cannot be separated from the person or exist independently. The term life-world attempts to express the complete "inter-relatedness or mutual dependence" (Valle & King, 1978, p. 10) between the person, the context, and the phenomenon. This world receives its significance from the acts of meaning that constitute everyday life. Individuals interpret these acts, and it is this collective interpretation that gives meaning to the phenomena. The lifestyle is an inherent part of this life-world.

Phenomenology attempts to represent an individual's conscious and/or mental experiencing of the world. "The primary emphasis is on the phenomenon itself exactly as it reveals itself to the experiencing subject in all its concreteness and particularity" (Giorgi, 1971, p. 9).

Consciousness is regarded as a "making present" where phenomena are revealed. In other words, consciousness always has an object. "It is by consciousness that objects are made present (are 'intended'); yet, equally as true, it is by objects that consciousness is revealed or elucidated" (Valle & King, 1978, p. 14). This process involves the *ego* (the self), the *cogito* (conscious activity), and the *cogitatum* (an object toward which conscious activity is directed, including physical objects and non-physical objects such as theories, other selves, moods, values). The process is represented as *ego-cogito-cogitatum*, in which the dashes between each word serve to point out that one is never present without the others. The self, conscious activity, and object exist together and represent human reality (Stewart & Mickunas, 1990).

One of the recognized founders of phenomenology was Edmund Husserl. Husserl (1960) believed that phenomenology could be used to provide descriptive truths about experience.

> *Because universals are rendered present in consciousness, Husserl believed it quite possible to reach objective knowledge (of whatever matter at issue, including things in the world as well as the human experiences of them themselves) by reflecting upon these universal structures and describing faithfully what appears. What makes phenomenology in principle possible is that in our ordinary conscious living, along with our apprehending the particular instance (e.g., a bicycle), we are also aware of the larger notion of what the instance is an instance of (e.g., bicycles in general). (Harper, 1981, p. 119)*

APPLICATION OF PHENOMENOLOGY TO THE LIFESTYLE PERFORMANCE MODEL

The process of phenomenology attempts to make explicit what is already implicit for individuals regarding the experience being studied. One way for this to happen is through personal descriptions of the lifestyle. Giorgi (1997) describes this as "a detailed concrete description of specific experiences from an everyday attitude from others" (p. 243). In addition, phenomenology requires that the description include reflection about the meaning of the lifestyle.

As an individual provides a description of his or her lifestyle, the practitioner must avoid letting personal views or beliefs about the nature or meaning of the experience of this individual's lifestyle influence the process. This involves "bracketing" of assumptions by the practitioner and presumes that the practitioner must first make them explicit in order to explain and understand their existence. "It seems that as one brackets his or her preconceptions, more of these emerge at the level of reflective awareness" (Valle, King, & Halling, 1989, p. 11).

The descriptions of conscious experiences are viewed as representations of the lifestyle. The practitioner recognizes the description as a lifestyle through common essences (invariants or constants). "It was, for Husserl, these invariants or constants—the ways human beings experienced the world—which he thought must be thematized in reflection" (Harper, 1981, p. 121). Within the Lifestyle Performance Model these essences include the process of being occupied, the activities that are the focus of the occupation, the real and symbolic meaning of the activities, and the environments. This brings a unique occupational perspective to the description of lifestyle. Husserl believed that there are many types of invariants or constants recognized at various levels. These range from individual, though typical, to universal. This search for occupational essences represents a crucial component of the phenomenological method.

The practice of occupational therapy from a phenomenological perspective requires the practitioner to set aside presuppositions about an individual's lifestyle. A conversation must be created that allows the individual to share his or her story using the concept of ego-cogito-cogitatum. The individual is viewed as expert regarding his or her knowledge of lifestyle. However, the concept of the individual is an "ensembled" perspective in which the self-other boundary is fluid in nature, control is contextually determined, and the person's conception of self is inclusive in nature, hence the concept of "lifestyle satisfying to self and significant other" (Fidler, 1996, p. 140).

The experience of occupational therapy within the Lifestyle Performance Model becomes discovery-oriented. The aim of the experience is to ascertain meaning, not to focus upon facts. Phenomenological questions revolve around the meaning and significance of occupational lifestyle for the participant, significant others and the practitioner. This implies that what is being sought is "what is really going on in" this lifestyle and "focusing on understanding the experience... from the multiple realities that coexist" (Hartrick, 1998).

The Lifestyle Performance Model has been built and modified based upon the notion of dynamic systems, non-linearity, and self-organization consistent with the theories known as *chaos theory* and *complexity theory*.

CONCEPTS AND PROPOSITIONS

The first chapter of this book provided an overview of the model and described a central construct (lifestyle) and sub-constructs (the four domains, the environments). Further, it stated that the outcome of using the model in occupational therapy practice was the enhancement of the quality of life of a person or population. The model is visualized using the metaphor of a spider web, as depicted in Figure 3-1. The strands of the web represent the inter-relatedness of the concepts and illustrate the dynamic nature of a lifestyle. As such, the lifestyle described at one point in time may be different than one described later in life. Like a spider web, the relative size of any one part varies depending on the environments and the actor.

WAY OF ORGANIZING

Because of the phenomenological basis of the Lifestyle Performance Model, a visualization of the structure that represents the model as heterarchal is crucial. In a heterarchy, no one part can totally represent the whole and no one part has more power than another. In the case of a lifestyle, a change in any part of a person's lifestyle (one of the domains, an aspect of the environment, a component of the individual) affects other portions. There is no direct, linear relationship regarding any changes that may occur. The flow of energy that maintains a

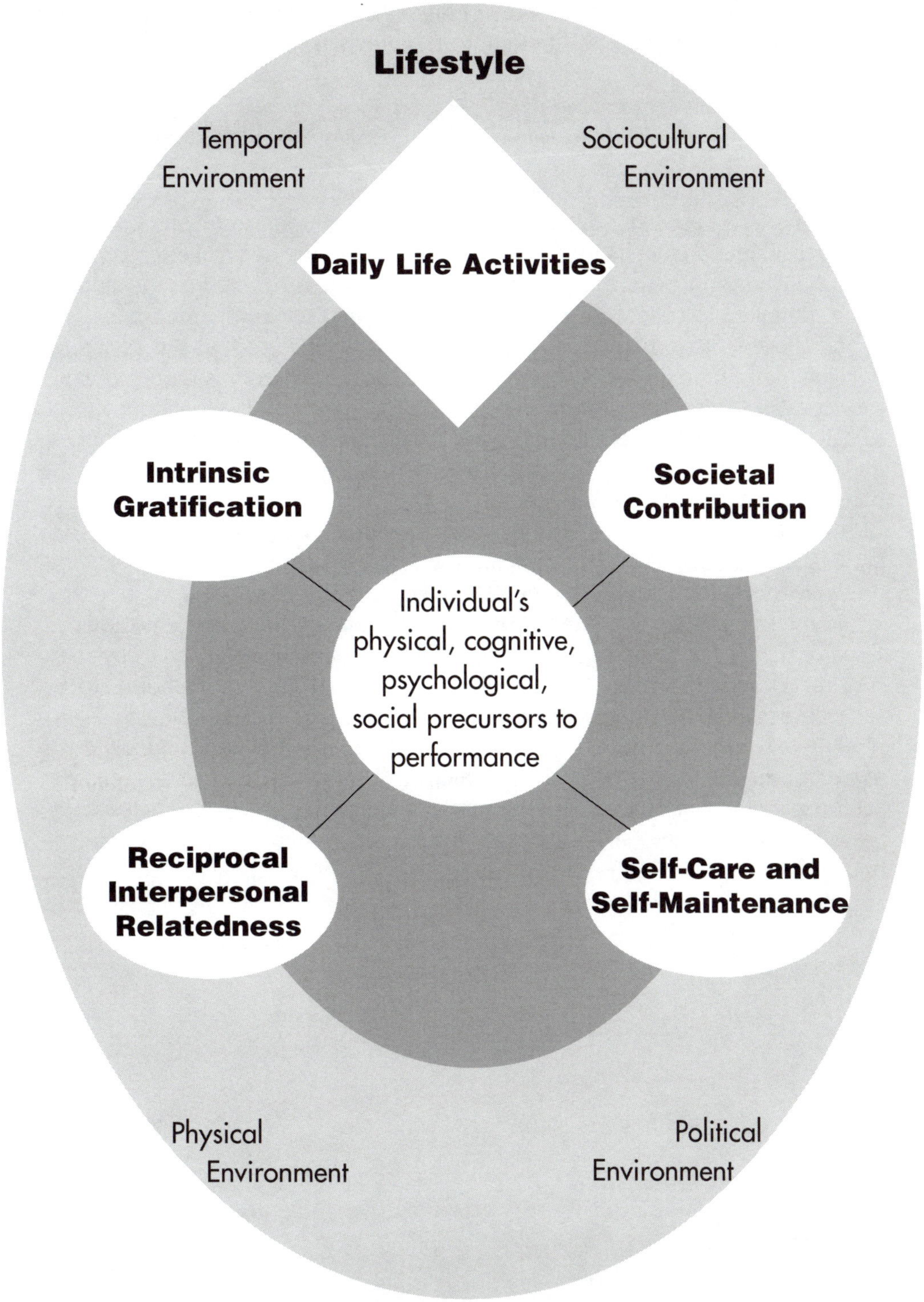

Lifestyle

Temporal
Environment

Sociocultural
Environment

Daily Life Activities

**Intrinsic
Gratification**

**Societal
Contribution**

Individual's
physical, cognitive,
psychological,
social precursors to
performance

**Reciprocal
Interpersonal
Relatedness**

**Self-Care and
Self-Maintenance**

Physical
Environment

Political
Environment

Figure 3-1. The lifestyle web.

lifestyle creates disturbances that are not predictable. The result may be a lifestyle configuration that is radically different from a previous one.

RESEARCH AND THE LIFESTYLE PERFORMANCE MODEL

As a theory grounded in the philosophy of phenomenology, research regarding the model is based in grounded theory and ethnographic traditions. Grounded theory is an interpretive method using both inductive and deductive reasoning to interpret data and build theory. Using grounded theory methods, the authors have continued to collect data, conduct analysis, and relate their interpretations to the Lifestyle Performance Model. Maintaining awareness that the continued development of the theory is grounded in the data, the theory is modified when new constructs emerge from the data generated. Reviewing the literature written to date about constructs of the model will provide the reader with an idea of how the method has influenced the model's development. This text summarizes the product of this grounded theory research.

Ethnography is currently being used to further investigate the Lifestyle Performance Model. "Ethnographers approach the field armed with theory... and, therefore, turn their attention to the culture within the framework from a particular theoretical perspective" (Stern, 1994, p. 215). Using ethnographic techniques, researchers have used the central construct of the model (lifestyle) and its five sub-constructs (the four domains and the environment) to study intact cultural groups such as occupational therapy student cohorts and community-dwelling elders residing in North Carolina (see Chapter 10). After collecting data from individuals regarding the constructs and sub-constructs, the researchers try to describe the culture from the perspective of the model. The outcomes of this research include articulating how the model in its current form does or does not fit designated cultural groups.

KEY POINTS

- Model of practice refers to a theory that is broad in nature and contains concepts or constructs and sub-concepts or sub-constructs.
- Frame of reference refers to theories of a more specific nature.
- Postulates describe the nature of the relationships between constructs and sub-constructs.
- Because of the phenomenological framework of the model, the primary research methods used at this time are grounded theory and ethnography.
- The sub-constructs include the four domains.

REFERENCES

American Occupational Therapy Association. (1997). The psychosocial core of occupational therapy position paper. *Am J Occup Ther, 51*, 868-869.

Fidler, G. (1996). Lifestyle performance: From profile to conceptual model. *Am J Occup Ther, 50*(2), 139-147.

Frank, L. K. (1968). Science as a communication process. *Main Currents in Modern Thought, 25*, 45-50.

Giorgi, A. (1997). The theory, practice, and evaluation of the phenomenological method as a qualitative research procedure. *Journal of Phenomenological Psychology, 28,* 235-261.

Giorgi, A. (1971). Phenomenology and experimental psychology: I. In A. Giorgi, W. F. Fischer, & R. Von Eckartsberg (Eds.), *Duquesne studies in phenomenological psychology* (Vol. 1, pp. 6-16). Pittsburgh, PA: Duquesne University Press.

Harper, W. (1981). The experience of leisure. *Leisure Sciences, 4*(2), 113-126.

Hartrick, G. (1998). A critical pedagogy for family nursing. *J Nurs Educ, 37*(2), 80-84.

Husserl, E. (1960). *Cartesian meditations: An introduction to phenomenology* (D. Cairns, Trans.). The Hague: Martinus Nijhoff.

Kielhofner, G. (1995). *A model of human occupation: Theory and application* (2nd ed.). Baltimore, MD: Williams & Wilkins.

Kielhofner, G. (1992). *Conceptual foundations of occupational therapy.* Philadelphia, PA: F. A. Davis Co.

McColl, M., & Pranger, T. (1994). Theory and practice in the Occupational Therapy Guidelines for Client-centred Practice. *Canadian Journal of Occupational Therapy, 61*(5), 250-259.

Miller, R. (1993). What is theory and what does it matter? In R. Miller & K. F. Walker (Eds.), *Perspectives on theory for the practice of occupational therapy* (pp. 1-12). Gaithersburg, MD: Aspen Publications.

Miller, R. J., & Walker, K. F. (1993). *Perspectives on theory for the practice of occupational therapy.* Gaithersburg, MD: Aspen Publications.

Morse, J. M. (1989). *Qualitative nursing research: A contemporary dialogue.* Rockville, MD: Aspen Publications.

Morse, J., & Field, P. (1995). *Qualitative research methods for health professionals* (2nd ed.). Thousand Oaks, CA: Sage.

Mosey, A. C. (1992). *Applied scientific inquiry in the health professions: An epistemological orientation.* Rockville, MD: American Occupational Therapy Association.

Nelson, D. (1997). Eleanor Clark Slagle lecture: Why the profession of occupational therapy will flourish in the 21st century. *Am J Occup Ther, 51,* 11-24.

Stern, P. N. (1994). Eroding grounded theory. In J. M. Morse (Ed.), *Critical issues in qualitative research methods* (pp. 212-223). Thousand Oaks, CA: Sage.

Stewart, D., & Mickunas, A. (1990). *Exploring phenomenology* (2nd ed.). Athens, OH: Ohio University Press.

Straus, A., & Corbin, J. (1990). *Basics of qualitative research: Grounded theory procedures and techniques.* Newberry Park, CA: Sage.

Valle, R. S., & King, M. (1978). An introduction to existential-phenomenological thought in phenomenology. In R. S. Valle & M. King (Eds.), *Existential-phenomenological alternatives for psychology* (pp. 6-17). New York, NY: Oxford University Press.

Valle, R. S., King, M., & Halling, S. (1989). An introduction to existential-phenomenological thought in psychology. In R. S. Valle & S. Halling (Eds.), *Existential phenomenological perspectives in psychology: Exploring the breadth of human experience* (pp. 3-17). New York: Plenum Press.

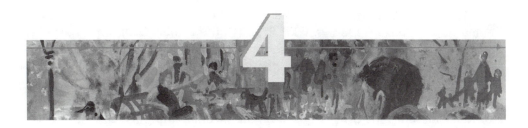

The Four Domains

An activity which is *purposeful* and *meaningful* to the individual contributes positively to that individual's perception of his or her own quality of life (Asker, 1990; Hoover, 1992; Sinnott-Oswald, Gliner, & Spencer, 1991; Wehman, 1993). Activities attain personal meaning through voluntary engagement of the individual's mind and body in the pursuit of an end goal that is relevant to personal needs, interest, capacities, and fulfillment of one's life roles (Fidler, 1994). According to Fidler (1996),

> An inherent belief underlying the model is that quality of life is the single most important theme in human performance. That wellness and a sense of well-being are understood as a state of being that is optimally satisfying to self and to significant others. It is hypothesized that such satisfaction is gleaned from personally and socially relevant activities that focus on and maximize individual strengths, capacities, and interests. Most important is the concept that intrinsic motivation is elicited and sustained when there is congruence between the characteristics of an activity and the biopsychosocial characteristics of the person. (p. 140)

Activity that is meaningful to the individual implies that the individual has had some experience with the activity. Meaning is established by "the perceptual sense it makes to the individual as well as to the cognitive associations elicited in the individual" (Nelson, 1988, p. 635). Through the actual "doing" of an activity, the individual understands or makes sense out of the experience and remembers the experience by integrating his or her cognitive, affective, and psychomotor responses to the activity. Activities may also be purposeful to the individual when the activity will assist the individual in meeting a stated or unstated goal(s). The individual interprets the activity based on the meaning that has been developed through past experience and its relationship to its potential for meeting a more future-oriented goal.

Many authors discuss activities in two essential categories: work and leisure (Day, 1985; Barnes, 1990; Brown, Bayer, & Brown, 1988; Glyptis, 1989; Clark & Hirst, 1989). However, with the changes in lifestyle created by employment patterns, technology, and the economy, viewing activities from this dichotomous relationship may be less useful than in the past. Instead, activity can be described through its relationship to the experiences a person has every day. Fidler (1996) proposes four grouped areas depicting the reasons a person uses to describe engagement in the activity and why it is meaningful to him or her. These are: self-care and self-maintenance, intrinsic gratification, societal contribution, and reciprocal interpersonal relatedness.

Our research of the Lifestyle Performance Model over the past 5 years has involved extensive data collection from more than 225 individuals using qualitative methodology. Through the Lifestyle Performance Interview, information about the four domains has been collected from university and college students, inmates, community-dwelling elders, individuals hospitalized with chronic unipolar depression, and children with their families. We have included in the following descriptions of each domain examples of activities and concepts developed from our research.

The research has also supported and enhanced our understanding of the propositions discussed in the first two chapters of this book. For example, the research supports the idiosyncratic nature of the domains insofar as each individual will place activities within the domain based upon his or her interpretation of their meaning. The placement of the activities within domains appears to change as the person progresses through different life stages. Finally, many individuals placed the same activity in more than one domain.

SELF-CARE AND SELF-MAINTENANCE

Activities that involve meeting one's personal needs in a manner that is self-dependent fall within the domain of self-care and self-maintenance. Self-dependence is not the same as independence. In self-dependence, the individual is able to recognize and articulate his or her personal needs so that, if unable to complete the task independently, someone is able to assist him or her when given direction. Research participants describe activities of personal care as toileting, bathing, dressing, eating, and grooming. Research participants frequently include sleep as an activity of this domain, although the level of engagement is very different than the other activities listed.

Self-maintenance activities involve functional activities of daily living. These include behaviors required to live independently in the community such as use of the telephone, food preparation, housekeeping, laundry, shopping, money management, transportation, and medication management.

Participants in the research of the Lifestyle Performance Model clearly recognize self-care and self-maintenance activities, and the data supports a common perception of activities as described above. Participants suggest that an awareness of one's own wants and needs enhances satisfaction with activities in this domain. They also imply that independence is an expectation of Western society, and people who are independent in self-care are valued more highly than those who need assistance.

This is not the perception of self-maintenance. Receiving assistance in activities commonly perceived as self-maintenance is acceptable and, for some, a designation of higher sociocultural status. Examples given included hiring a house cleaner or driver, purchasing food prepared in a restaurant, hiring a nanny for child care, and using investment consultants for money management.

Reasons given for alterations across a life span of the activities placed in this domain are frequently related to developmental changes such as changes in role (becoming a parent and adding child care activities), changes in physical status (changes in vision resulting in the loss of a driver's license and subsequent need for help in grocery shopping), or changes in housing type (such as movement from a family home to retirement home, minimizing activities of yard maintenance).

SOCIETAL CONTRIBUTION

Activities contributing to the need fulfillment and welfare of others fall within the domain of societal contribution. Based upon the interviews, activities include paid work, volunteer experiences, and education or other activities in which a service is provided to others. Research participants talked about the ability to recognize needs and wants in others as necessary to choosing activities in this domain. They described the relationships within this domain as more unidimensional, with little expectation of reciprocity. In other words, they engaged in these activities to serve the needs of others. Occupational roles filled within this domain were not always those that were intrinsically gratifying to the research participant. Examples of these roles included server, disciplinarian, and cleaner.

RECIPROCAL INTERPERSONAL RELATEDNESS

Activities pursued in order to develop and sustain relationships with others and that involve reciprocity fall within the domain of interpersonal engagement. Perhaps more than any other domain, occupations here depict what Moore and Anderson (1968) describe as activities of strategy. They are activities in which all actions and outcomes are influenced and determined by the interplay of two or more people. Unlike the area of societal contribution, research participants expect a give and take between participants, often suggesting a 50:50 split. Research participants discuss relationships involving peers, friends, family, and acquaintances. The activities involve sharing secrets, writing letters and emails, talking on the telephone, meetings around food, family events, and one-to-one conversations. The strength of the bond is important to the research participants, and it is the quality of the relationship–not the quantity of relationships–that enhances satisfaction with this domain. As one research participant stated, "I am satisfied in knowing that if I needed one of them, he would be there for me just as I would for that person."

INTRINSIC GRATIFICATION

Activities that an individual pursues because of the pleasure and enjoyment they offer to the individual fall within the domain of intrinsic gratification. Typical activities described by research participants included playing or attending sports, attending cultural events, reading, participating in fitness activities, and going on vacations.

Research participants acknowledged that satisfaction in this domain requires a clear understanding of their own wants and needs regarding fun and enjoyment. Further, active attempts to satisfy these needs and wants must be achieved without guilt. Some participants discussed balancing planned activities with spontaneous decisions. Others mentioned the eight elements of enjoyment further described by Csikszentimihalyi (1990) as being essential for an activity to be described as intrinsically gratifying.

One concern raised by research participants is that activities described as intrinsically gratifying are often the first to be eliminated when there is a lack of time or money. One set of research participants, elders residing in a rural community strongly bound by religion and family, had difficulty naming activities identified as intrinsically gratifying. One of the reasons given by these participants for this difficulty was the strong cultural influence of service to others.

BALANCE OR HARMONY?

When considering quality of life from an activity perspective, it is natural to wonder if individuals require an equal distribution of activities in each domain with similar amounts of time spent in each. This would be considered by many to represent balance. This balance could be measured at one point in time and over a lifetime. Within the area of leisure, authors also discuss the need for balance in the type of activities (such as sports, culture, entertainment) and level of participation (such as active or passive) (Austin & Crawford, 1991; Peterson & Gunn, 1984; Howe-Murphy & Charboneau, 1987).

When the concept of activities is broadened to represent four areas that are not mutually exclusive, the quantitative concept of balance does not fit. An alternative is the concept of harmony, in which the number of activities or amount of time spent in each domain does not have to be equal. Instead, each domain is related to the others, but the focus is upon the individual's perception of "a pleasing arrangement or combination of parts" (Morehead & Morehead, 1981, p. 249).

Data analysis indicates that one link between activities and the individual's perception of harmony is *continuity*. Continuity includes maintaining some activities across the individual's lifetime. Often, while the activity remains part of the person's repertoire, the type of participation changes. For example, one individual may begin as a player of a sport, move to the coach, then become a spectator, and finally watch the sport on television. Participants also discussed being in control of their own activity repertoire, making decisions for themselves about the level of participation and type of activities to include. A third component of harmony revolves around the ability to engage in the activities that match the participant's own value system. When the activity repertoire is represented to self and others (those personal values described as critical to the person's self-image), then the lifestyle is more likely to be perceived as harmonious.

THE USE OF ANALOGY

The inter-relationships of the four domains and the environment are complex. One way to understand the model itself is to liken the model to an object, a story, or a process. Many participants in the Lifestyle Performance Study have been asked to write or verbally describe the model in this way. These descriptions have portrayed the model as a hamburger sandwich, a tree, a home, a space shuttle, a tire and wheel, a flower, and the sun. What follows is an edited description of one participant's understanding of the model using the analogy of a growing tree. The author of the analogy is a woman and consequently the pronoun "she" is used throughout:

> *A seed is planted into the ground. Here it derives minerals and other essentials to grow. But, it cannot grow by the soil alone. Rainwater must seep through the soil and reach the seed as well. The seed soon develops many roots, which are forever part of the tree.*
>
> *As the seed, now a tiny tree, breaks out of the ground, it rises upward slowly. It is different from the ground, though nourished by it, and different than the grass and stones. Yet, all of these things are part of the tree's environment. The tree grows branches and unto these branches,*

more branches. It sprouts leaves, and sometimes the leaves change color or fall off. Many people can tell what type of tree it is by its leaves, the number of leaves, and whether the tree loses its leaves.

Over the years the tree has grown and changed. It has been nourished by the soil through its roots and by the rain. The tree now has many ridges on its trunk, with some being deeper than others. These give the tree character. A few branches have broken off in a storm, others have grown solid and strong, while others have decayed and been replaced by new branches. Many seasons and storms have occurred. The tree is still growing.

A person, like a seed, begins her life implanted in a culture (soil). The culture influences every part of her early life from assigning roles, to establishing values, and most importantly influencing beliefs and perceptions. The influences of culture are received through socialization, through others. The roots formed represent these: the family, friends, neighborhood, and religion. The roots are the earliest and strongest influences in a person's life and are what will continue to fuel a person's growth throughout life. They are the foundation for what the person will hope to achieve, what she views as being good, who she will become as an individual, what she chooses to do, and how she will interact with others.

Just as some roots on a tree are bigger than others, some roots in the person's life may be a larger influence. For example, if the person's family is troubled, she may rely on interpersonal relationships, religious activities, or community involvement. I began this analogy by talking about a seed. Most cultures would designate the origins of the seed as being from some higher power and having a spirit. The spirit of the seed, like the spirit of the person, is nourished by the higher power, represented as the rainfall.

The seedling breaks through the ground and begins to fully become separate and different. This is the point in each person's life where she begins to become autonomous to the degree valued by her own comfort and cultural roots. It is a unique balance where comfort and familiarity of one's roots are distanced from a person's striving for a sense of self-differentiated from others. While the roots are always part of the tree, the tree continues to grow taller and more defined as it interacts with the environment.

To survive, the seedling differentiates itself from other parts of the soil environment. The human also defines herself as different from her roots and as being related to, yet different from, other objects in her physical environment. She is different than an inanimate object, yet objects serve as a means to express herself, to help forge relationships, or provide a sense of mastery. Objects hold much value, but the value is often only recognized when the object is gone.

The tree develops many ridges on its trunk, and its trunk grows larger and taller. The core of the trunk represents the precursors the person needs to engage in activities—neurologic, psychologic, physical. The ridges symbolize the traits of the individual: personality, desires, goals, likes, dislikes. These individual traits are partially shaped by the cultural roots and partly shaped by the interaction with the environment. Experiences, engagement in activities, are filtered through the environment and cultural roots to become part of the person's activity repertoire or not.

The tree begins to grow branches and leaves. The branches represent the active part of the person's life, with the vast repertoire of skills learned through exposure to the environment. Every branch comes from one of the four main branches formed out of the trunk. They are connected to the individual, and each represents areas where a person chooses to concentrate activities: service to others, intrinsic gratification, reciprocal interpersonal relatedness, and self-care/self-maintenance.

The smaller branches represent activities, and the leaves on the branches represent specific tasks within activities. They are dependent on the branches (skills in domain) to be able to accomplish them. They are also dependent on the environment to support them. If a leaf is not well supported, it decays and crumbles away. So too, if a task is not done to the person's satisfaction or society's, the person may cease to be engaged. This happens whether the cause lies within the person (precursors) or the environment. Just as there are many types of tasks in each domain that change across the person's life span, the leaves on the tree change colors as the tree ages.

The individual uses beliefs and her own psyche to form perceptions. Perception is like the outer surface of the tree—under the bark. It develops from the roots, the core, to interact with the environment. Perception is used to rate all experiences, the individual's success and failures in activities, to re-evaluate cultural roots, and to develop a fundamental view of health. Perception in turn determines levels of motivation, beliefs about health and quality of life, and reactions to activities and people. To assess quality of life, the person's perceptions must be tapped.

KEY POINTS

- The four domains are sub-constructs of lifestyle.
- The domains are self-care/self-maintenance, intrinsic gratification, reciprocal interpersonal relatedness, and societal contribution.
- An activity may represent more than one domain.
- Individuals strive for a sense of harmony among the domains.
- Harmony is composed of continuity, control, and match to values.
- Activities within the domains take place in a variety of environments.

REFERENCES

Asker, D. (1990). *The interdependence of leisure activity and cultural values.* ERIC Document Reproduction Service No. ED 320889.

Austin, D., & Crawford, M. (1991). *Therapeutic recreation: An introduction.* Englewood Cliffs, NJ: Prentice Hall.

Barnes, C. (1990). *'Cabbage syndrome': The social construction of dependence.* New York, NY: The Falmer Press.

Brown, R. I., Bayer, M. B., & Brown, P. M. (1988). Quality of life: A challenge for rehabilitation agencies. *Australia and New Zealand Journal of Developmental Disabilities, 14*(3/4), 189-199.

Clark, A., & Hirst, M. (1989). Disability in adulthood: Ten-year follow-up of young people with disabilities. *Disability, Handicap & Society, 4,* 271-283.

Csikszentimihalyi, M. (1990). *Flow: The psychology of optimal experience.* New York: Harper Collins.

Day, H. I. (1985). A study of quality of life and leisure. *Rehabilitation Digest, 16*(2), 102-106

Fidler, G. (1996). Lifestyle performance: From profile to conceptual model. *Am J Occup Ther, 50*(2), 139-147.

Fidler, G. (1994). Foreword. In C. Christiansen, (Ed.), *Ways of living* (pp. v-vi). Baltimore, MD: American Occupational Therapy Association.

Glyptis, S. (1989). Leisure and unemployment. In E. Jackson & T. Burton (Eds.), *Understanding leisure and recreation: Mapping the past, charting the future.* State College, PA: Venture Publishing Co.

Hoover, J. (1992). Development of a leisure satisfaction scale for use with adolescents and adults with mental retardation: Initial findings. *Education and Training in Mental Retardation, 27,* 153-160.

Howe-Murphy, C., & Charboneau, B. (1987). *Therapeutic recreation intervention: An ecological perspective.* Englewood Cliffs, NJ: Prentice Hall.

Moore, O. K., & Anderson, A. R. (1968). *Some principles for the design of clarifying educational environments.* Pittsburgh, PA: University of Pittsburgh, Library Learning Research and Development Center.

Morehead, A., & Morehead, P. (1981). *The new American Webster handy college dictionary: Revised and expanded edition.* New York: Signet Book.

Nelson, D. (1988). Occupation: Form and performance. *Am J Occup Ther, 42,* 633-641.

Peterson, C., & Gunn, S. (1984). *Therapeutic recreation program design: Principles and procedures* (3rd ed.). Englewood Cliffs, NJ: Prentice Hall.

Sinnott-Oswald, M., Gliner, J. A., & Spencer, K. C. (1991). Supported and sheltered employment: Quality of life issue among workers with disabilities. *Education and Training in Mental Retardation, 26,* 388-397.

Wehman, P. (1993). *The ADA mandate for social change.* ERIC Document Reproduction Services No. ED 354660.

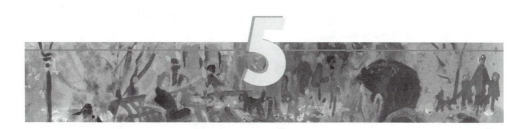

The Environmental Context

An environment can maximize performance to the extent that it includes, emphasizes, and ensures by nature of its structure, operations, philosophy, and interpersonal practices those doing experiences—those activities that optimize *autonomy, individuality, affiliation, volition, predictability, self-efficacy, adventure,* and *reflections*—from the perspective of human performance.

The needs, interests, and concerns of a society are, in many ways, portrayed in the environments it creates for its own use. Each of these entities (e.g., the school, home, industry, hospital, community center) consists of a number of inter-related components designed and set in operation to achieve the purpose of its existence. The most commonly acknowledged components of these society-created environments typically include those structures and processes that relate to communication, decision making, design and use of space, furnishings, fiscal management, social relationships, time management, custodial/housekeeping, and external affiliations. While these functions seldom vary in kind among environments, there are significant differences in how they are carried out and in the priority assigned to them. The structural and procedural methods that are characteristic of an environmental component clearly reflect the philosophy, beliefs, and attitudes of the organization of which it is a part. For example, the structure and operations of a school will reflect beliefs and attitudes about how learning occurs and about expectations regarding students and teachers. A nursing home's management of time and fiscal allocations is most frequently a statement about the philosophy regarding chronic care and aging.

It would therefore certainly be misleading to attempt to describe environmental components without consideration of those factors that influence how they function. The characteristic qualities, the ambience of an environment and its components, are a complex inter-relating mix of social, cultural, economic, and political dynamics. The inter-relationship among these elements is evident in a variety of ways and commonly accepted as a reality. For example, political agendas as well as cultural values frequently influence fiscal management and allocations. The distinction between the two influences is seldom possible. Recent debates about how our education system should be structured reflect an intriguing mix of social, cultural, political, and economic factors.

The intertwining of self, society, and environment is expressed by Yandell (1995): "We create our immediate environment and then contemplate it and are worked on by it. We find ourselves mirrored in it, see what had been not yet visible, and integrate the reflection back into our sense of self" (p. xiv).

POLITICAL ENVIRONMENT

Society's values and interests are reflected in its regulatory acts, laws, ordinances, and rules. Those acts that govern hospital and nursing home standards, schools and educational systems, social behavior, health care systems, accessibility, and nature of care have a decided impact on the shaping, the operations, and the use of person-created environments. Such regulations evolve from sociocultural values and beliefs, from political interests, and from economic values and concerns. School systems across the country differ in standards and regulations regarding, for example, inclusion or segregation of students with disabilities. Therefore, the environments within which teachers and special service professionals function, as well as how they may practice, vary accordingly. How decisions are made and how and what is communicated then differ in relation to local regulations and their integral values and beliefs. Likewise, nursing home regulatory standards differ between states, reflecting cultural values, and economic and political dynamics. In response, the role of the occupational therapist in terms of communication and decision-making behavior, interpersonal relationships, and time management will vary in accordance with the given environment.

In another context, family values, cultural heritage, and political and economic orientations, of course, have a marked influence on how a household functions and how they relate to one another and to its broader community environment. These include both implicit and explicit rules. What gets talked about within the family and with whom, the nature and frequency of external affiliations, how decision making is handled, and patterns of spending and saving are only a few examples of how such dynamic variables create an environment and influence its components. These are very critical considerations in developing an individual Lifestyle Performance Profile.

TEMPORAL ENVIRONMENT

Individuals, groups, and societies orient themselves to many types of *time* such as mechanical, personal, inner or psychological, natural, and social. Mechanical time is the type to which we most commonly refer. It describes an orientation to the seconds, minutes, hours, and 24-hour day. Practitioners use mechanical time as an outcome measure of performance, as a delineator of treatment time, as a workday, and as a determination of discharge.

Personal time refers to the biophysiological aspects such as circadian rhythm or circummensual. Practitioners need to take into consideration the sleep-wake cycle, natural periods of alertness, and female cycles in planning and conducting occupational therapy programming.

"I never have enough time" and "time flies" are examples of inner time. Frequently tied to the person-occupation congruence, this type of time affects motivation, attention, and participation by influencing the person's perception of how participation in the occupation matches his or her expectations.

The day-night light cycle, seasons of the year, and cyclic view of time held by many cultures is referred to as natural time. This type of time impacts performance and participation in many ways. For example, elders may decrease engagement in activities outside the home at night because of fear or difficulty seeing in the dark. Specific seasons of the year facilitate certain types of activities—winter skiing and summer swimming. Air conditioning has changed neighborhood activities—people stay inside versus sitting on stoops or porches. Cold weather limits outside activity for many, including limiting walks, gardening, etc., and substituting indoor activities such as watching television.

Social time refers to those periods of the day and night when members of the same cultural group have a common understanding about time use. For example, it is easy to tell lunch time in most places of employment and educational institutions by observing behavior and activities. Similarly, families develop activities oriented to social time such as bed times relating to age and family role, specified meal times, and family television time. Social time appears to be somewhat artificially regulated and controlled by customs of the dominant culture.

THE PHYSICAL ENVIRONMENT

The physical environment is viewed as the context, "the setting" in which human endeavor occurs. The environmental contexts are most frequently acknowledged as including those entities, those settings created by persons and by nature. People-created entities include homes, communities, institutions, organizations, and agencies. Nature-created settings include wilderness areas, waterways, green spaces, and the like.

Humans create environments for their own use, for survival, and for the development and maintenance of society. Homes, schools, community centers, pharmacies, churches, hospitals, restaurants, and nursing homes each have their purpose in being and each comprise a variety of activities designed to achieve their reason for being. Spivak (1973) adds to these classifications by including environments that are created for the purpose of attending to emotional needs such as churches, temples, museums, parks, and mountain trails. Clearly, natural environments are protected and used in terms of persons' interests, needs, and values. The activities that occur within each setting are influenced by the nature or characteristics of that setting. Parks, green space, waterways, and backyards all provide the opportunity for unique occupations and for bonding with nature. For some, these spaces allow for nurturance—the phenomenon of "Mother Earth." For others, they provide adventure and the potential to overcome fear of the spiders in the woods, the dark and damp spaces harboring untold danger.

There are those environments oriented to mobility such as skiing, canoeing, or hiking; securing food such as fishing or hunting; or risk such as climbing or caving.

The natural environment offers a challenge of coping by managing the natural elements such as heat, cold, rugged terrain, darkness, turbulent waters, and wind. By contrast, man-made environments offer the challenge of coping and adapting to the rituals, performance requirements, and ambiance of the setting. These realities are critical in terms of the model's focus on the congruence of occupational engagement and human needs and interests. The compatibility between a person's abilities and interests, the environment itself, and its performance requirements is an important dimension of successful performance and sense of achievement. This aspect of intervention goes beyond treating the individual for performance deficits that limit use of the man-made environment, or ensuring physical access to the building or adaptation of the physical objects within the structure. This person-environment congruence also includes ensuring each individual a place for privacy, a place for association with others, variable degrees of order in the environment, a means for expression of autonomy, and a means for expressing individual needs such as self-efficacy.

Fidler and Bristow (1992) suggest that those environments created by society can be understood as having two major functional dimensions. One relates to the physical qualities of design and structure. The other embodies interpersonal structures, procedures, and relationships—the human aspects of operations related to the sociocultural environment. Each one is characteristically different but necessarily integrated to form the total character meaning and function of the whole. Both the functional realities of these environmental components and their symbolic statement are of critical importance for understanding and facilitating human performance (Fidler & Velde, 1999; Fidler & Bristow, 1992).

There is ample evidence that *space* influences human behavior. Over-crowded classrooms are seen as impeding learning and giving impetus to disruptive behaviors. Rioting and aberrant actions in prisons are most frequently attributed to overcrowded space and related problems. By contrast, it has been noted that large open spaces can be disturbing and experienced as cold, unfriendly, and impersonal. Each person has what might be called his or her own special comfort zone related to one's neuropsychology and culture. Hall's (1966) intriguing study of the relationships between space and human activity supports this thesis. His research demonstrated the relationship between spatial distances and interpersonal engagement. He further substantiated the hypothesis of varying cultures defining spatial comfort differently.

Clearly, space is a noteworthy variable in consideration of the congruence of the person-environment equation. In facilities, the allocation of space will most frequently reflect the assigned value and priority of the activity or service. Entitlement to an office or assignment to a congregate area; allocation to ground floor, top floor, or underground space are indications of priorities and preference. The importance of personal space is evident in a variety of settings.

Small cubicles of desk space in congregate areas are most frequently adorned with personal objects and photos. Nursing homes encourage residents to personalize space with their special mementos and objects. Ownership of personal space in the home is clearly made evident by the banners and trophies of the teenager, and in another space the treasured objects of parents (Csikszentmihalyi & Rochberg-Halton, 1981). Activities that support and help to clarify "my-space," "your-space," "our-space" are valuable, especially in the home and in extended care environments. For example, in one setting patients contributed the paintings and drawings they had made for the dining area, signifying our-space. In another, a group of residents were engaged in creating objects and photo displays for their rooms that would signify my-space. In a different context, Fidler (2000) describes the neighborhood project of creating our-space for shared activities.

The *ambient elements* of an environment such as light, sound, color, and temperature have a marked effect on performance. We are aware of the studies that relate the type and intensity of light power to hyperactivity of the student with attention deficits. As well, there is the noted influence of light on an individual's circadian rhythm and sleep-wake cycles. The placement and intensity of lighting is an important concern in facilities that care for the aging. Color is a closely related element, and one can find a number of studies and speculations about the effect of color on human and animal behaviors. Some studies, for example, have suggested that the use of warm colors such as oranges and deep pinks seems to reduce aggressive behaviors in prisons. The warmer colors are more readily distinguished and thus aid in visual orientation for elderly and visually impaired persons.

Speculations regarding the symbolic significance of color are many: the intense blue signifying power, the purple of royalty, and the ubiquitous yellow tie of corporate America a decade or so ago. The effect of the combination of color and space on behavior was evident in a facility providing care for persons with Alzheimer's disease. The refurbishing of the activity area had created a room with bright ceiling lights, off-white walls, and floor tiles. Although staff considered it "cheerful," patient behaviors of disorientation, confusion, and agitation escalated. Painting the walls a contrasting warm mauve had a markedly positive effect.

Sound is an additional element that contributes to the ambience of an environment. As our world becomes more diverse, more crowded, and complex, its sounds likewise are more varied and intense. "Deadly silence" and "auditory overload" are expressions reflecting extremes. Determining what may be a facilitative level and kind of sound for a given setting requires thoughtful attention. It has been noted, for instance, that a certain kind of music tends to increase worker productivity as well as student attentiveness and learning. In contrast, the silence of fans at a sporting event seems to reduce the competitive drive of their athletes. Each of us at one time or another has experienced annoyance with the noise in a restaurant that interferes with conversations. In congregate settings, it is difficult for individuals to control or adjust sound or other sensory input. Turning off one's hearing aid in response to sound overload is an acknowledged practice. However, this action then diminishes conversation and engagement with others. The significance and value of adapting environmental elements became evident in an initiative involving nursing home residents. The lack of mealtime conversation was notable, although in other settings many residents did engage verbally with others. When the background music and the sound of an adjacent television were turned off, when the wheels of the serving cart were muted and tables reduced in size, conversation and exchanges with others emerged.

The type and placement of *furniture and equipment* has a direct influence on the performance and behavior of individuals and groups, as well as impacting the operations of a total environmental entity. For example, the efficiency of computers and their accessibility is well known. The ready availability, supply and use of books and other learning equipment and resources, and the arrangement of classrooms determine the efficacy and limitations of a school. The roles of family members, the nature and frequency of their interpersonal engagement is certainly influenced by the equipment, the furnishings of the kitchen, the living room, and other spaces in the home. The placement of furniture in the waiting rooms of medical services environments is an efficient use of space but serves to reinforce the kind of behavior that is expected. When these are arranged in a circle or semicircle to enable eye contact, social exchange is more likely. For the elderly, chair arms and firm cushion seats are acknowledged as important for use and mobility. Attending to and influencing the arrangement of an area to facilitate achievement of the goal of intervention is an important responsibility of a practitioner.

COMPONENTS OF THE SOCIOCULTURAL ENVIRONMENT

The *social* and *interpersonal* components of an environment are significant determinants of its functional effectiveness and reflect its character and related feeling tone. The nature of family member relationships–child, parent, sibling, and those persons outside the family group–are acknowledged factors in defining and reflecting personal performance expectations, philosophy, values, and sense of satisfaction. Likewise, the school, the rehabilitation center, the service agency, or the nursing home that includes in its policies and procedures opportunities to engage in activities that foster a sense of belonging; having a stake in the enterprise; of being included, recognized, and valued is an environment that maximizes human endeavor, motivation, and satisfaction.

Closely related to the interpersonal dynamics of an environment is the component that comprises *communication*. Who talks to whom and about what? Who is privy to what kinds of information and its sharing? What information and topics get shared (e.g., only between parents, among management, or other clusters)? How is information gathered, shared, or disseminated? In what ways do patterns of communication reflect a sharing-discussion process or "telling" dissemination? How are gossip and rumors handled? These are only a few issues and concerns which, when addressed, will shape and reflect the characteristics of a given environment and significantly impact its functioning and those who have a role in fulfilling its purpose.

How *decision-making* is perceived and implemented and who gets to make which decisions are critical questions in the operations of any planned environments. How decisions are handled in a family, school, hospital, or community reflects philosophies, values, and beliefs about management, parenting, subordinate-superordinate roles, human behavior expectations, and collaboration. Decision-making and communication policies and processes are significant influences on the practice of occupational therapy. What information is readily available, from whom, and what are the traditional patterns of collaborative sharing and assessment? What information should be shared with the client, with the client's family? Furthermore, what decisions is the practitioner empowered to make and under what circumstances? What constitutes autonomy and responsibility in solo practice as compared with a practice with an agency or facility? Clearly, these concerns and how they are handled shape the kind and nature of intervention decisions.

Fidler and Bristow (1992) suggest that clarification of "the what" and "the who" in decision-making is a critical dimension of this process. They propose addressing three questions in the quest to understand the what and who of decisions (pp. 31-32):

1. What decisions can I make on my own without necessarily consulting anyone?

2. What decisions must I make in collaboration with others and with whom?

3. What decisions are beyond my control, influence, and expertise?

An example of using components of the sociocultural environment identifies the marked change in the atmosphere of an assisted living facility. A transformation occurred when two occupational therapy students created an activity called "Food Around the World." A group of residents and staff were supported in exchanging recipes, preparing, and serving their culturally varied foods. Communication barriers between staff and residents began to diminish, tensions lessened, and relationships began to be more relaxed. Excursions into local communities were initiated by the group to learn about different cultures and, for a few residents, even a renewal of interest in food.

AN ENVIRONMENTAL PROFILE

The structure and functioning of an environment and its complex, interacting components both shape and reflect the character and behavior of individuals, communitles, organization, and societies. From the perspective of the Lifestyle Performance Model, environmental influence is manifested in the kind of activities or occupation that characterizes a given setting. The model further contends that the extent to which the setting-specific activities are congruent with fundamental human needs is a significant measure of the quality of life within that setting. Therefore, a principle concern of the model is to explain and enhance the roles of activities in defining, shaping, and reflecting the characteristics of a given environment and to maximizing the relationship of each to satisfying human performance and the quality of life. This mission can be addressed in part by developing an environmental profile that will:

- Identify the commonly acknowledged components of a given environment.
- Describe the characteristics of the activities that comprise each component.
- Relate these patterns of activities to requisite human needs.
- Describe additions and/or alterations regarding activities that could be expected to enhance the relevance with human needs as well as support the purpose of the environmental entity.

Relevant information about each environmental entity can be gathered from a variety of sources, including on-site observations, interviews with persons involved within or using the setting, document reviews such as philosophy and mission statements, operating policies and procedures, annual reports and other records. Interpretation of data is used in several ways.

At an individual level, the concern is to identify and describe what activity alterations and/or additions could be made to maximize personally gratifying and rewarding personal engagement. For example, the occupational therapist working with persons who are homeless may advocate activities for housing and habitat as well as involve the individuals in a variety of tasks related to building or refurbishing available living space. In addition, this practitioner might also use the data to develop opportunities for personally relevant activity engagement related to the four domains of the model within the structure of the homeless shelter, thereby enhancing the shelter environments as well as the daily life experience of its members.

GATHERING INFORMATION ABOUT THE ENVIRONMENT

At an organizational or systems level, an occupational therapist might work to decrease tension and increase collaboration by organizing a staff-client music combination in a forensic hospital or data interpretation might be used to ameliorate communication problems by organizing a student-teacher newsletter group that would replace the more formal top-down memos and bulletin board notices. A first concern of the environmental profile is to describe those activities that are an integral part of a given environmental entity. In essence, to describe those actions, those doing experiences, which comprise, for example, a school's communication system or a households' meal activities. Fidler and Velde (1999, pp. 157-158) have identified 11 environmental components, and the following guidelines for gathering information related to these is adapted from their work.

1. **Communication:** What are the activities that relate to the information-gathering and dissemination processes? Who are the committees, clusters, groups, and/or persons involved in creating and disseminating information such as newsletters, flyers, and documents? What activities include the informal networking, the procedures of passing along inside information and gossip? In a household, these activities might include discussions over supper intended to catch up on members' activities, recording messages, or writing letters.

2. **Decision-making:** What are the activities that incorporate the processes of discussing, critiquing, and recommending decisions through such venues as family caucuses, student government, advisory boards, boards of directors, executive councils, labor representatives, supervisors, and managers?

3. **External networking:** What activities represent and enable affiliations with outside organizations, groups, and individuals such as churches; political, civic, and welfare associations; public education systems; and volunteering organizations?

4. **Facility care and management:** What activities relate to the care and maintenance of the physical space inside and outside of the facility or home? These might include cleaning, trash removal, bed making, heating, lighting, and maintenance of safety, furnishings, and interior decorating.

5. **Food management:** What activities relate to the planning, preparation, serving, eating, and clean-up of food? This includes the joint efforts of individuals, task forces, committees, and groups concerned with the planning of menus for special occasions, addressing member preferences, and evaluating food-management activities.

6. **Fiscal management:** What long- and short-term planning activities completed by groups, committees, and/or individuals are related to planning and budgeting, allocations, monitoring, and purchasing policies necessary for the survival of the environment and its constituents and members?

7. **Furnishings:** What activities relate to the consideration of the impact of furnishings on the nature of activities; the acquisition and placement of furniture and decorations; displays of personal objects, diplomas, trophies?

8. **Person relationships and management:** What activities signify belonging, such as formal and informal planning and carrying out of special ceremonies, events, team sports, trips, picnics, and retreats? Other examples include acknowledgment of participation in activities such as citizen of the

year awards, honor roll achievement, elected office, gaining special privileges, and life review. Committees that relate to the development and monitoring of personnel policies, member roles, and responsibilities frequently conduct these activities.

9. **Space utilization:** What activities are concerned with the planning, allocation, and use of space? This component Includes the description of the impact of space on member performance and operational activities such as conferences, committee meetings, small and large group activities, privacy, and social events.

10. **Time management:** What activities reflect the involvement of members in planning and carrying out the schedules of daily living activities such as rising; grooming; meal time; weekday/weekend distinctions; holiday times; free time; day, evening, and night time schedules?

11. **Political:** What activities reflect the implicit and explicit rules of society regarding engagement in the occupational process?

Based on this information, an analysis is undertaken to discern the nature of the relationship between the activity experiences and human needs. Such a comparative analysis explores the nature and frequency of opportunities for members of the environmental entity to experience autonomy, individuality, affiliation, volition, consensual validation, predictability, self-efficacy, adventure, accommodation, and reflection (Fidler & Velde, 1999).

It should now be possible to note what additions and changes could be made to the activity components that would enhance the relationship of an environment's functional activities to human needs and simultaneously strengthen and sustain the purpose of the environmental entity. What activities might be added, for instance, to the communication process that would enhance the sense of affiliation or volition? For example, when an assisted living facility was plagued by numerous and persistent complaints about food, a resident food committee was formed to work with the dietary department. This resulted in a marked reduction in complaints and improved residents' eating patterns. Most significantly, it resulted in a shared collaborative effort and feeling. Reduced neighborhood tensions and other positive changes resulting from activity opportunities that addressed human needs have been noted by Fidler (2000). Fidler and Bristow (1992) offer significant evidence of the positive impact when organizational activities are congruent with human needs. The title of their book, *Recapturing Competence*, is in fact a statement of outcome when organizational behaviors are restructured to match human needs.

The Lifestyle Performance Model views the environment as a critical dimension to understanding human performance in an effort to enhance quality of living. It should be eminently clear that attention to this dynamic and the environmental profile are essential for implementing the model.

KEY POINTS

- Environments both support and constrain occupation.
- Environments demand participation in a set of activities.
- Environments include the political, temporal, sociocultural, and physical.
- Data gathering for the purpose of intervention planning includes information about the environments.

REFERENCES

Csikszentmihalyi, M., & Rochberg-Halton E. (1981). *The meaning of things: Domestic symbols and the self.* Cambridge, England: Cambridge University Press.

Fidler, G. S. (2000). Beyond the therapy model: Building our future. *Am J Occup Ther, 54,* 99-101.

Fidler, G. S., & Bristow, B. (1992). *Recapturing competence.* New York: Springer.

Fidler, G. S., & Velde, B.P. (1999). *Activities: Reality and symbol.* Thorofare, NJ: SLACK Incorporated.

Hall, E. T. (1966). *The hidden dimension.* Garden City, NY: Doubleday.

Spivak, M. (1973). Archetypal places. *Architectural Forum, 140,* 48-50.

Yandell, J. (1995). Foreword. In C. C. Marcus (Ed.), *House as a mirror of self* (pp. xiii-xvi). Berkeley, CA: Conari Press.

Data Gathering

Conducting the Lifestyle Performance Interview

Since the Lifestyle Performance Model comprises two major areas of concern—the person-lifestyle configuration and the environmental context of performance—the data-gathering processes for each will, of course, differ. This chapter deals with the content, focus, and procedures concerned with defining and obtaining information that will make it possible to design an individualized activity-based lifestyle configuration. Those data-gathering initiatives related to the environmental context of the model are explored in Chapter 5.

Approaching the task of data gathering requires keeping in mind the fundamental orientation of the model. The model is a personalized, subjective approach to "the what," "the how," and "the why" of an individual's engagement in those activities that comprise that person's daily living routines. It is based on the belief that the person's quality of life is a result of the interplay between the characteristics of the person, his or her activity choices, and the sociocultural values of that person's environment.

LIFESTYLE PERFORMANCE PROFILE

Data-gathering processes that are most relevant to the Lifestyle Performance Model use methodologies that engage the person in reflecting on and developing his or her story about what has been, what is, and what might be the activity patterns that comprise his or her living and the meaning of these for self and significant others. The aim of gathering such data is to enable a collaboratively developed, activity-based lifestyle performance profile that is as personally and socioculturally relevant as possible. This information then serves as a template, a guide toward working to achieve a satisfying, productive lifestyle. When a person is unable to communicate directly with the practitioner, methods other than a personal interview are imperative. Such methods could include observation, interviews of significant others, discussion with other health providers, and formal/informal preference assessments.

Such collaboration involves a partnership between the practitioner and the occupational therapy participant (hereafter called the participant) in order to develop descriptions of:

- What is and what has been the person's daily living activity patterns in each of the model's four domains. It includes the individual's personal preferences relative to these domains.

- The attitude of the person regarding these activity patterns.

- The self-other relevance of these. That is, how these patterns fit or do not fit with the needs, interests, and capabilities of the person and the values and expectations of that person's social matrix.

- Current performance skills, strengths, and limitations in each domain within the context of the self-other satisfaction equation.

- Family and community sociocultural values in relation to each domain.

- Existing geographic, economic, sociocultural, and legal resources and limitations in the immediate environment.

- Individual characteristics (e.g., physical, psychological, cognitive), capacities, and attitudes that shape performance.

- The harmony, balance-imbalance among the domains within the context of age, environmental expectations, and the dictates of personal capacities.

LIFESTYLE PERFORMANCE INTERVIEW

The personal interview is clearly the preferred method for data gathering in the Lifestyle Performance Model, and the Lifestyle Performance Interview has been developed to address the information needed to implement the model. For those readers who are unfamiliar with the semi-structured and unstructured interview techniques recommended for administration of the Lifestyle Performance Interview, a suggested reading list is provided at the end of this chapter. Based upon the responses gathered during the Lifestyle Performance Interview, the practitioner may gather additional information using standard occupational therapy instruments to assess one or more performance components. The outcome of the process is the development of a Lifestyle Performance Profile that is unique to that individual.

The Lifestyle Performance Interview, when skillfully managed, comprises an open-ended dialogue that nurtures the subjective reflection and personalized perspectives so necessary to design a personal lifestyle profile. This process, similar to any other interpersonal engagement, encompasses two spheres of communication, the verbal and non-verbal. Non-verbal communication is the silent language, the messages embodied, for example, in body posture and movements, eye contact, facial expressions, tone of voice, and choice of physical setting and its ambiance. The practitioner is simultaneously engaged in monitoring her or his own non-verbal communication and attending to that of the participant. For example, positioning of the extremities could reflect an openness or closedness to the interview, postural congruence between the practitioner and participant might suggest empathy, and gestures can support the conversational tone of the interview. Sensitive reactions to facial expressions of both self and the participant can facilitate an attitude of trust and interest.

THE INTERVIEW'S SETTING

Organization of the physical setting should promote comfort and privacy for both parties. Attention to the site chosen for the interview is essential. For example, conducting the interview in the participant's room or home offers the opportunity to note objects and furnishings that elaborate on the participant's lifestyle. Alternatively, asking the participant to choose the site empowers him or her regarding the process.

Since most interviews are conducted while seated, the practitioner should weigh the advantages and disadvantages to using a table. Consideration of where the participant should sit in relationship to the practitioner is also essential. Sitting next to the person conveys a different message than sitting across from the person. Many times, a set-up in which the chairs are at 90 degrees offers a solution to concerns about power messages, ability to maintain eye contact, and maximizing hearing acuity.

These silent messages speak of values, attitudes, expectations, self-regard, confidence, comfort, and anxieties. Since non-verbal communications have a significant impact on the interviewing process and its outcome, it is important for the person conducting the Lifestyle Performance Interview to continually work toward enhancing awareness of self and one's comfort with others.

Verbal communication is just that. It is the use of language, language structure, and form to communicate. Gathering meaningful data is most apt to occur when questions and comments are open-ended and exploratory. Questions that can be answered in one word, such as yes or no, inhibit reflection and limit exploration. Those asking "what do you think" rather than "why or how do you feel" are considerably more facilitative since they are less apt to elicit a defense.

ETHICAL PRINCIPLES

To maintain the ethical principles of the interview process, participants have the right to refuse to answer any question and to terminate the interview at any time. This guarantees the right to privacy. Participants also have the right to confidentiality. To accomplish this, both should have an agreement that articulates who has access to the data gathered. Finally, the written information and/or audiotapes need to be kept in a secure place, and common agreement regarding their disposition at the end of the intervention process must be reached.

Listening skills, being able to objectively hear what is being said, are a critical factor in an interview. Preoccupation with obtaining adequate data or formulating questions, or a general anxiety about managing well, limits the ability to truly listen. Practicing active listening skills such as restatement, reflection, and clarification is an important dimension of enhancing interviewing skills.

Tape recording of the Lifestyle Performance Interview offers several advantages. It preserves the full content of the engagement and allows the process to supercede content. The practitioner can gain clues to his or her strengths and needs regarding interviewing skills by listening and reflecting upon the tape. It furthermore avoids the pitfalls of note taking, such as overlooking some material, selective hearing, and/or preoccupation with the note-taking process itself.

A comfortable, productive interview is, in the last analysis, reliant on interpersonal knowledge and skills. The suggested reading listed at the end of this chapter offers opportunities to refresh and enhance such know-how. Furthermore, it must be remembered that interviewing skills improve with practice and reflective critique.

COLLABORATION

The intent of the Lifestyle Performance Interview is to gather information about a person's lifestyle. The practitioner and participant are partners in the process on an equal level. The practitioner has expertise in this method of data collection while the participant is the content expert, with knowledge of his or her lifestyle. To be a true artist, the practitioner must maintain an attitude of naiveté regarding the individual's lifestyle, approaching the interview with assumptions and preconceived biases held in abeyance. Rapport and a beginning sense of trust can be developed when the practitioner shares information about self, is responsive to critical cues, and reflects an attitude of interest. Further, by being responsive to changes in spoken words, intonation, persistent responses, unusual words, and behavioral characteristics, the practitioner can organize the format of the Lifestyle Performance Interview to enhance the quality of the data collected.

INTERVIEWING PITFALLS

Typical pitfalls while conducting the interview include discomfort with silence, limited skills in handling silence, being too directive, following suggested questions too closely, difficulty in coping with expressed emotions, and staying on the topic. The development of skills to cope with these is done through experience, self-reflection, review of audiotaped or videotaped interviews, and solicitation of feedback from those who are more skilled in the process.

In the initial stage of the Lifestyle Performance Interview, several tasks must be included. Guidelines for conducting the interview need to be established. These include ethical principles such as issues of privacy and confidentiality, practical issues such as breaks and interruptions, role expectations of the practitioner and participant, time limits, and an explanation of how/where the interview fits in the intervention process.

QUESTIONING

The primary focus of the Lifestyle Performance Interview is to gather information about a person's activity patterns within each of the model's four domains. The following material offers suggestions for gathering data about each domain. The practitioner needs to evaluate and select questions that will contribute to the knowledge needed to develop an individualized lifestyle profile. While examples of questions that are appropriate for various age and cultural groups and a variety of occupational and life roles are offered, the questions adopted must be individualized by the practitioner after consideration of the participant. This can be difficult if this is the first encounter between the two. However, the practitioner can gain data about the individual from many sources, including data provided by other professionals, information from family and significant others, medical and social service records, etc. Questions are used to facilitate reflection and responses, not to obtain "a correct answer" or establish facts.

The quality of the responses may be enhanced by probing or following a response with a question of clarification or elaboration. The questions can be reworded to fit the needs of the interview situation. Phrasing probes as a follow-up to the initial question may help in getting quality responses. Some examples are "Can you tell me about…" "Do you remember an occasion when…" "How did you…" or "Are there other examples?" Frequently, during responses to questions about one domain, the participant may provide data about another domain. The practitioner should note this and refrain from repeating requests for information previously provided.

The practitioner needs to be flexible and maintain the conversational quality of the interview. There are many ways to begin the Lifestyle Performance Interview. For example, the interview might follow a chronological sequence—addressing a person's lifestyle across a life span, problem-solutions order, describing changes and transitions in a lifestyle, movement from simple to complex concepts—or begin with the interpersonal and move to the personal. The practitioner's preparation regarding the content and focus of the interview requires an in-depth understanding of the Lifestyle Performance Model. This allows for a dialogue with clear expectations and data that is usable in constructing a lifestyle profile. Most practitioners who use the Lifestyle Performance Interview find it useful to complete a self-profile before using it to gather data from another individual.

CONSTRUCTING A PROFILE FOR A NON-VERBAL INDIVIDUAL

What happens when the person cannot be interviewed directly because of lack of communication skills or influence of a health condition? In this case, the practitioner must get to know the person through alternative means. These might include:

1. Spending time with the person to observe likes and dislikes.
2. Conducting informal and/or formal preference assessments.
3. Interviewing friends, family, and caregivers.
4. Observing the person's environments and his or her reaction when in them.
5. Noting significant objects in the personal environment and the person's interaction with them.

During observations, the intent is not to analyze the person's occupational performance but to gain an understanding of the occupations in the participant's lifestyle and to note those that appear satisfying.

When depending on other persons' interpretations of the participant's communication, the practitioner needs to be aware that miscommunications occur in the interpretation process. The practitioner must evaluate how adequate the others' skills are in the interpretation process. As Brown, Gothelf, Guess, and Lehr (1998) state, "caregivers… rely on their own interpretation of an individual's non-symbolic, idiosyncratic, inconsistent, or self-selected modes of communication (e.g., vocalizations, gestures, and facial expressions)" (p. 19). To verify the interpretation, practitioners should gather cumulative and comprehensive information from a variety of sources about the participant's lifestyle.

LIFESTYLE PERFORMANCE INTERVIEW

Self-Care and Self-Maintenance

Exploration of this domain will reference those tasks and activities that are routinely carried out as one's chosen patterns of personal hygiene, health care, grooming, and dressing. It also encompasses those chosen activities concerned with feeding self, money management, clothing self, household management, living in the community, and travel.

Occupational therapy literature offers an abundance of material related to this domain. These publications provide a wealth of information that delineates and describes the constructs and procedures for evaluating and treating dysfunction related to self-care. The over-riding focus in most of the literature is on defining and remediating pathological and dysfunctional self-care behaviors. However, there are some exceptions to this circumscribed orientation. For example, Christiansen (1994) and Fidler and Velde (1999) emphasize the multi-dimensional aspects of self-care, viewing its inter-related activities as a self-narrative that expresses a personal identity, social orientation, and sociological and cultural values.

The Lifestyle Performance Model views self-care and self-maintenance from such an orientation. Activities in this domain are explored as reflections of personal needs, interests, and characteristics; interpersonal orientations; and sociocultural values, attitudes, and ethics. As noted, the repertoire of activities and attendant attitudes that comprise this domain, as well as the other domains, are considered from such perspectives. Thus, the focus of the data-gathering interview is to build a narrative of a person's self-care and self-maintenance activities and the meaning these have for the person and significant others. The following questions are offered as interview guides. They are adapted from Fidler and Velde (1999, p. 119). There are no mandates regarding the sequence or their total inclusion. Questions should follow the natural unfolding of a dialogue and seek to facilitate its qualitative nature.

Self-Care

What are those activities that you use to care for yourself? How are they organized? Are you satisfied with those activities? Are you satisfied with your performance of those activities?

Probes

Describe your daily routine upon arising each morning.

How much time do you spend each morning grooming and dressing?

How does this routine vary on weekends and holidays?

Do you shower or tub bath? What is the difference for you?

Do you use a mirror? For what purpose?

What factors do you consider when deciding what to wear?

How is your grooming and dressing alike or different from your peers, parents, colleagues, or others?

What is most important to you in terms of your attire and grooming?

continued

For whom do you dress and groom?

How do you shop for clothes? Do you shop alone? With a friend? How often? Is it planned or spontaneous? What type of stores do you shop?

What opinion do you think others might have regarding your style of dressing and grooming?

Considering all that is involved in these activities, what do you find most enjoyable? Least enjoyable? Dislike?

Are you satisfied with your ability to care for yourself? In what ways?

Do you experience any difficulty in managing the tasks of personal hygiene, grooming, or dressing? What are these?

Would you like to make any changes in this aspect of your daily life?

Management of Living Area

What activities do you do to manage your living space? How are they organized? Are you satisfied with those activities? Are you satisfied with your performance in those activities?

Probes

Describe the household furnishings item that is most important to you.

What objects in your home have very special meaning for you? In what ways?

What factors influence you most in furnishing your living space: color, style, comfort, utility, other?

In what ways are your furnishings and living space alike and different from your friends, your parents?

Which household tasks do you perform regularly? What influences your choice of these?

Which ones do you enjoy? Dislike? Avoid?

Are there homemaking tasks that are difficult for you to manage? In what ways?

How would you describe your housekeeping style? Neat and tidy? Casual? Untidy?

How were household tasks managed by your parents? Who was responsible for which tasks?

How were you and your siblings involved in household maintenance?

Of these—outside space, lawn, garden—which are a regular responsibility? How are these tasks managed? Which are enjoyable for you? Which do you dislike?

continued

How were these tasks managed by your parents?

Do you share living space with another? If so, how are your housekeeping styles alike? Different? How do these affect your relationship? How do you share/divide tasks?

If it were possible, what changes to this area might you like to make?

Food and Eating Patterns

What activities are part of eating and food preparation? How are those activities organized? Are you satisfied with those activities? Are you satisfied with your performance of those activities?

Probes

To what extent do you engage in meal planning and preparation?

How frequently do you eat out? Eat alone? With others?

Do you share cooking, meal planning, eating with another/others? Describe.

How important is food to you?

Do you shop for food? What is that experience like for you?

Are there tasks related to obtaining, planning, and eating food that you find enjoyable? Describe. Are there some you find a chore or not enjoyable? Describe.

Who did the cooking, shopping, and related tasks in your family?

How would you describe your mealtime routines and behaviors? For example, regularity, casual, sit down "family style"?

What are the most difficult or problematic parts of your present meal preparation and/or eating? How do you manage these?

Money Management

What activities do you do to manage your money? How are they organized? Are you satisfied with those activities? Are you satisfied with your performance of those activities?

Probes

Do you manage your own finances?

How would you describe your typical style of managing your money?

How do you set spending priorities?

When money runs short, what is your usual way of approaching the problem?

continued

How is this like or different from your peers, your parents, others?

Is planning for your future needs important to you? If so, have you developed and followed through on a plan?

Health Management

What activities reflect the way you manage your health? How are they organized? Are you satisfied with those activities? Are you satisfied with your performance of those activities?

Probes

How much attention do you pay to your health?

What do you do regularly to maintain your health?

Do you consider yourself to be an active or sedentary person?

How do you describe your health-related activities and preference?

How health conscious was your family when you were growing up?

Societal Contribution

This domain comprises those tasks and activities that have as their primary purpose contributions to the welfare and need fulfillment of others. They are done for the contribution, not because any reciprocity is expected. The process of gathering information related to this domain explores those activities that shape and signify a sense of self as a productive, participating member of one's society. The process explores the person's activity patterns that are viewed as necessary to the survival and well-being of others. This includes the nature and personal meaning of one's social roles, such as wage earner, homemaker, parent, student, community member, volunteer, and the like. The following questions are offered as guides for the interview:

What activities represent wage earning? How are they organized? Are you satisfied with those activities? Are you satisfied with your performance of those activities?

Probes

Describe your current primary career or job.

How did you come to make this choice?

Have you had previous wage-earning experiences? What have these been like?

What is the most enjoyable aspect of your present career or job?

What do you like least about it?

What are the most difficult parts of your current career or job?

continued

What skills do you have that are important for you present career or job?

Do you expect this choice to be a long-term commitment for you? If not, what are your long-term goals?

How would you assess your skills for this choice?

To what extent do you enjoy what you are now doing?

How would you describe the kind of person you think it takes to do well in your present (and/or future) career or job? How well do you fit that description?

How would you describe your choice in terms of its complexity, supervision given and received, extent of routine and detail, problem-solving responsibilities, decision-making responsibilities, job pressures, job security, compensation such as salary/bonuses, awards?

How important do you think your career or job is to society? To your family? To friends?

If you could change any aspect of your career or job, what changes would you make?

What percentage of weekly time do you spend in your career or job activities?

How different or alike are your free time activities from your primary career or job?

Considering all aspects, what does your primary career or job choice mean to you?

What non-wage-earning activities do you do that contribute to the well-being and needs fulfillment of others? How are they organized? Are you satisfied with those activities? Are you satisfied with your performance of those activities?

Probes

As a student, which subjects do you or have you enjoyed the most?

What are/were your grades in these?

Which subjects do you/did you dislike? What are/were your grades in these?

How does your role as a student contribute to the present and/or future needs of others?

What volunteer activities have you and are you presently engaged in?

What do you find most satisfying about these?

How are these like or different from those of your peers?

Are there other activities that you do to help others such as your family, friends, school, church, and community?

Intrinsic Gratification

This domain is concerned with those activities that are devoted to personal pleasure and enjoyment—those activities performed for the sheer pleasure in the doing. The interview will explore the person's choices of such activities and their meaning to the individual in terms of the dimension of personal enjoyment and sense of pleasure. The following questions are offered as guides for the interview:

What are the activities that you do simply for fun and personal pleasure? How are they organized? Are you satisfied with those activities? Are you satisfied with your performance of those activities?

Probes

Which of these do you find especially enjoyable? What is special about them?

What other activities would you like to explore?

What gets in your way of such pursuits?

In terms of enjoyment, which of the following do you enjoy more:

Being an active participant or participating as an observer?

Competitive or cooperative activities?

Activities done alone or as part of a group effort?

Indoor or outdoor activity?

Free, expressive activities or those with more structure, guidelines, and directions to follow?

To what extent do your activities include sports, games, art, crafts, other? How frequently are you involved in each?

In what ways are your current activities like or different from those of your childhood?

What relationships do you see between the activities that you pursue for fun and those in other domains?

Considering all aspects, characterize your fun activities.

Reciprocal Interpersonal Relatedness

This domain encompasses those activities that have as their primary purpose the enrichment of one's relationships with others. Included in this domain are those activities that are shared with loved ones, family, friends, colleagues—those that embody group membership, belonging, and intimacy and that have in their nature elements of reciprocity.

What activities do you do because of the interpersonal relatedness included in those activities? How are they organized? Are you satisfied with those activities? Are you satisfied with your performance in those activities?

Probes

What activities do you engage in with friends? How frequently?

How are the activities important to your friendships?

What activities do you share with family members (spouse, significant other, parent, sibling, other relatives)?

What activities are shared together as a family group? How important are these to you?

What activities are characteristic of your intimate relationship?

What activities do you share with acquaintances, colleagues, co-workers?

What group activities and affiliations are part of your daily life (church groups, school, political, neighborhood, groups, etc.)?

What social events are part of your lifestyle? How frequently?

What is especially positive about them?

Which social activities do you dislike or prefer to avoid?

What activities with others do you remember from your growing up years as especially pleasant, unpleasant?

How would you characterize your pattern of activity engagement with others?

What changes would you like to make in these activity patterns?

Reflection

To bring closure to the Lifestyle Performance Interview, it is important to allow the participant time to reflect upon both the content and the process of the experience. This will also aid the practitioner in the interpretation of the wealth of data obtained. In addition, the Lifestyle Performance Interview session should close with the practitioner providing information about the next stages in the process, the estimated timeline, and the role of each participant and practitioner.

Summary Questions

1. After considering all aspects of your daily life activity patterns, which aspects or parts do you consider as being most important to you at this time? Which is of least importance?

2. What changes would you like to make?

3. How might you begin to bring about such changes?

SUPPLEMENTAL INFORMATION

It is expected that all Lifestyle Performance Interviews conducted within the context and focus of these guidelines will provide an adequate perspective of an individual's sociocultural values and orientations. Gathering information to construct a Lifestyle Performance Profile, including the interview, record review, observations, etc., can take between 1 and 2 1/2 hours to complete. The actual length of the interview depends upon the skills of the interviewer, the verbal abilities of the participant, and information available from other sources such as medical records, charts, and other professionals. The interview can be done across several shorter time segments when necessary. The practitioner is responsible for gathering the required materials including the tape recorder, tapes, power source, notebook for commentary, pens/pencils, and questions. The data gathered during the interview are supplemented with evaluations of performance components (when necessary), relevant data from other sources (such as records), observations (such as furnishings and objects in the participant's physical setting), and data regarding the environment (see Chapter 5). This should be sufficient to form the basis for developing collaborative recommendations and guidelines for a personally relevant Lifestyle Performance Profile.

Traditionally, performance components (i.e., those "building blocks" of performance behaviors) are viewed as priority concerns in occupational therapy theory and practice. The Lifestyle Performance Model certainly views these as important, however they are of secondary consideration in evaluating and building a Lifestyle Performance Profile. Assessment and evaluation of a component of performance is addressed only when it is demonstrated that a given component interferes with or precludes achieving a satisfying lifestyle from the participant's perspective or when it is expected that a clinical assessment of a given component will lead to more relevant and personally satisfying accommodations.

The standardized instruments and procedures chosen for assessing a component and defining a remedial process is a decision to be made by the practitioner. These instruments and procedures are represented in the various frames of reference common to occupational therapy practice. They include the cognitive, motor, physical, psychosocial, perceptual, sensory, and other systems of the body. There is a variety of credible options, and selection of an approach should be made on the basis of the practitioner's expertise. If additional information seems necessary regarding the social, cultural, economic, or political nature of the environment, then community demographics, social welfare agencies, and other community resources can be tapped.

In summary, the overall purpose of gathering information is for the client and practitioner to arrive at an understanding of the personal meaning of the person's daily activity engagements. From this, they determine if any alteration could or should be made to enhance the level of satisfaction for that person and for those who share in that person's living. This process of interpretation is discussed in Chapter 8.

KEY POINTS

* Data about the four domains is gathered using interview, observation, and consultation with other professionals and documents.
* A Lifestyle Performance Profile illustrates a person's occupational story.
* The profile identifies both strengths and needs regarding occupational performance.

REFERENCES

Brown, F., Gothelf, C. R., Guess, D., & Lehr, D. H. (1998). Self-determination for individuals with the most severe disabilities: Moving beyond chimera. *Journal of the Association of Persons With Severe Handicaps, 23*, 17-26.

Christiansen, C. (Ed.). (1994). *Ways of living.* Bethesda, MD: American Occupational Therapy Association.

Fidler, G. S., & Velde, B. P. (1999). *Activities: Reality and symbol.* Thorofare, NJ: SLACK Incorporated.

SUGGESTED READING

Denzin, N. K., & Lincoln, Y. S. *Collecting and interpreting qualitative materials.* Thousand Oaks, CA: Sage.

Fontana, A., & Frey, J. H. (1998). Interviewing: The art and science. In N. K. Denzin & Y. S. Lincoln (Eds.), *Collecting and interpreting qualitative materials* (pp. 47-78). Thousand Oaks, CA: Sage.

Egan, G. (1976). *Interpersonal living.* Monterey, CA: Brooks-Cole.

Fidler, G. S. (1982). The lifestyle performance profile: An organizing frame. In B. Hemphill (Ed.), *The evaluative process in psychiatric occupational therapy* (pp. 260-280). Philadelphia: F. A. Davis.

Pollio, H. R., Henley, T. B., & Thompson, C. J. (1997). Dialogue as method: The phenomenological interview. In H. R. Pollio (Ed.), *The phenomenology of everyday life.* Cambridge, UK: Cambridge University Press.

Stucky, N. (1995). Performing oral history: Story telling and pedagogy. *Communication Education, 44*, 1-14.

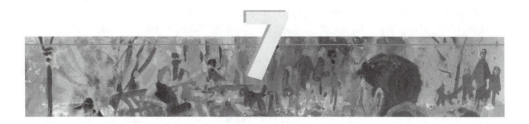

Examples of Lifestyle Performance Interviews in a Mental Health Setting

Michael Amory, MS, OTR/L and Beth P. Velde, PhD, OTR/L

The Lifestyle Performance Interview is a semi-structured interview based on the Lifestyle Performance Profile. Interdisciplinary documentation is incorporated when gathering data about the individual's lifestyle and precursors of performance. Individual observation is added to the information described in the profile as individuals are observed engaging in various purposeful activities.

A focused combination of interview and quantitative data (chart review, functional testing, individual observation, strength, and mobility testing) allows the occupational therapist to use various qualitative and quantitative data to understand the way of life of an individual. This flexibility is crucial to the occupational therapy approach as well as to the Lifestyle Performance Profile. Various occupational therapists (Estroff, 1981; Langness & Levine, 1986; Zola, 1982) have claimed that individuals with chronic physical or mental illnesses pose an ethnographic challenge to health care professionals. This is because conventional occupational therapy data-gathering processes such as standardized interviews or task observation may be useless, singularly, as the data gathered may not be rich enough to provide a holistic view. However, occupational therapists have the ethical responsibility of providing meaningful therapeutic activities based on thorough and accurate evaluation data. Therefore, the Lifestyle Performance Interview approach provides one way of knowing about the lifestyle of the individual with major depression—as discussed in this chapter—in a quick, comprehensive, and individually referenced format. This method allows the occupational therapist to use a vast array of data and data-gathering instruments to learn about the lifestyle of the individual.

LIFESTYLES OF PERSONS WITH MAJOR RECURRENT DEPRESSION

The following profiles represent individuals admitted to a psychiatric inpatient program where one must be over the age of 18, have a formally diagnosed exacerbation of an Axis 1 (DSM-IV) diagnosis, and be unable to function in a home situation either independently or with supportive services secondary to being a threat to themselves either directly through suicidal intent or indirectly through self-neglect.

The occupational therapist as well as other members of the professional staff (social worker, physical therapist, nurse, and psychologist) first evaluate the individuals. This information is obtained through interviews, records review, and family interview. It includes a social history, medical history, factors precipitating admission, family history, psychological history, treatment history, and a brief leisure history. From the initial assessment, the occupational therapists determine if the individual is able to tolerate and be amenable to a longer interview process. Such an individual needs to possess adequate verbal skills and openness to discussing his or her lifestyle. This may be supplemented with interviews of family/significant others as another means of gathering the interview data.

The individuals whose profiles are included seemed to enjoy the interview, as evidenced by their bright affect and thank you's at the end of each interview. In fact, Bonnie mentioned that the occupational therapist should do the interview with all of the patients, saying: "It makes you think... I've thought of some things I'm going to bring up in group." She went on to say that it made her remember things that she had not thought of for years, saying, "I think that some of the questions are behind the depression... I think they are deep; they are so far deep-rooted in you that you just kind of say, 'Aww, that isn't important.' Does that make sense?"

EILEEN'S LIFESTYLE PERFORMANCE PROFILE

Eileen is a divorced 66-year-old woman who has a long history of recurrent major depression with subsequent psychiatric admissions (a minimum of 10 times). She was admitted to the psychiatric unit voluntarily with symptoms of a depressed mood, suicidal ideation without a plan (a passive desire of not wanting to live), interrupted sleep, sense of loneliness, decreased appetite, and decreased interest in pleasurable activities. She identified three potential stressors: a strained relationship with her daughter who is not assuming household or child care responsibilities, change in medication, and chronic/ongoing problems with a respiratory cold. Eileen has had no admissions in the past 10 years and had been active in senior citizens' programs with aerobics and breakfast as late as 1 month ago, but has become less motivated to leave home or get out of bed recently. Her diagnoses included:

Axis I: Major depression, severe, recurrent, without psychotic features

Axis II: No diagnoses

Axis III: Good physical health

Axis IV: Moderate

Axis V: 40/80

Eileen was very reluctant to agree to the interview at first, stating that she wanted to "think about it" because it might drain her and upset her. She then finally agreed, stating, "If it will help you out I will do it." When she was informed about the tape recorder she hesitated and asked, "Can we do it without that?" but then acquiesced. During her first interview, her speech was slow and she frequently paused for long periods of time both after questions and during her answers. However, she was generally very open and did not appear uncomfortable with any of the questions. The Lifestyle Performance Interview was broken into two interview sessions. On the day after the first part of the interview, Eileen frequently asked, "When are we going to finish?" as if she was eager to speak with me again.

Societal Contribution

Eileen was a nurse in a large hospital. She experienced a lot of satisfaction helping sick people and stated, "I know just being a nurse I felt I had a purpose in life and after I took retirement, for a while it was hard for me to get myself together." She retired in February of 1985 on disability after 14 years as a full-time nurse. She hasn't "been doing that much [to help others] lately." Her primary avenue of serving others involves her live-in daughter and 2-year-old granddaughter. About this Eileen states, "She's there with a baby and I just feel I should stick around the house and help her." She has to pick up after her daughter, who she states will "get some juice out in the morning and drink half of it and let the other there, and she'll do the dishes and not really complete it." She also does much of the laundry for them and describes having to straighten up her room "like she is a little girl." It seems that she resents this service, as she states, "It's bad enough picking up after a baby but when you have to pick up after her..." She also describes being in charge of the flowers at church, although she states it "seems like a chore." Later in the interview she described wanting to get a part-time job as a nurse's aide in a nursing home but stated, "If they found out about my history then they wouldn't hire me."

It is important to note that the activities Eileen describes are those in which she does not expect reciprocity from the individuals involved. However, Eileen is quick to point out that societal contribution is typically acknowledged in some way. In her case, she has identified her perception of barriers to her performance in this domain. They include her medical history, society's perception of mental illness, and assisting her daughter with child care.

Reciprocal Interpersonal Relatedness

Eileen describes herself as having no close friends. Her main social outlets are church once a week where she is a choir member, the senior citizens center on weekdays, and belonging to a bowling league where she bowls once a month. Occasionally, she goes to movies or day trips with "an acquaintance." She repeatedly describes herself as feeling inferior to other people and states, "I'm such an inferior, I have an inferiority complex. I know that I have problems and I feel people can sense it." She has no one close to confide in and stated she would call the minister if she were afraid or needed help. She describes having a poor relationship with her daughter, though she wishes it were different. She states, "I wished there would be somebody who would be more forceful and just kind of sit there and take us apart and see what we're doing to each other. She describes her marriage as being a poor decision and claims that it was his parents who split them up. She said he was a kind man but states that "I guess maybe I didn't love my husband, but I know he loved me, so that hurt."

Self-Care and Self-Maintenance

Eileen independently runs her house, which she owns. She has money problems and feels she does not budget well. She likes to buy nice clothes but describes having difficulty shopping for clothes because she is short, stating, "I'm not always happy with the way I dress." Lately, she describes grocery shopping as an effort and she has difficulty knowing what to buy. In fact, at times she buys groceries and gets home and realizes that she doesn't have anything to make a meal. In addition, she dislikes and has difficulty with meal planning and preparation and states, "I make a mess; I have more dishes when I make anything... I don't like the disorganization of it. My whole house I feel is disorganized; it's an old house. I don't have a place for everything and anything in its place so it gets scattered around just like my mind." She likes to do minor repairs herself, as well as painting and small household jobs.

Intrinsic Gratification

Although Eileen has lost interest in almost all leisure activities, she describes one of her favorite activities as gardening and yard work, telling others, "I'm going to play in the dirt a little bit." She has a big yard and grows a couple of tomato plants, pepper plants, strawberries, and flowers, saying, "But when I'm out doing that I just don't seem to think about other problems." In addition, Eileen does "plastic crafts" such as knitting and crocheting. "I made a lot of afghans over the years, and now I got a new sofa and love seat and they're completely a different color than all of these afghans I made. Everything is like helter-skelter. You know, nothing matches, nothing goes together. I don't go together." Presently, she has stopped doing crafts because they are not enjoyable and stopped reading because she cannot concentrate. She mostly watches TV, including movies, documentaries, and news programs. Her only joyful experiences are times with her granddaughter. She is generally vague when describing childhood activities and replies, "I don't know, I don't remember," although she stated that bike riding was a favorite childhood activity.

Future

The therapist asked questions about her perception of her future. Overall, she has hope that she will do better once her daughter moves out. If she had her wish she would have a different, modern home in the country with private bedrooms for her two children and grandchild. She expresses a lot of negative feelings about her house, stating that she made a poor decision when she bought it and she's been paying for it ever since. She was doubtful if her future would be better but states, "Hopefully better, I'm not saying definitely."

Eileen would like to get involved with helping people again. She discussed possibly going back to working in a nursing home as an aide but expressed a lot of doubt about her ability to handle it: "I think of that from time to time, and when I'm feeling bad I think 'oh, how can I even do that; I'm just so tired'."

Personal History/Culture

Eileen could not choose one particular object that she thinks describes her, but she did say her crafts in general tell something about herself (i.e., afghans, plastic crafts, embroidering). "They show that I'm creative." She appeared to strongly identify with the role of a mother, saying, "I've always been the mother, planning meals, preparing clothes." However, she expressed regret that her children do not come to her for advice, saying, "They don't come to me for any advice, help... I want to be someone that—a mother that—my children can come to for any advice when they need. I seems to be they're hesitant to come and ask for help."

Eileen's favorite subjects in school were the humanities (i.e., biology, German, Latin). "That's because it was interesting and fun learning." Her least favorite subject was algebra. Eileen was vague when discussing her parents' and sibling's activities. She remembered going camping in the mountains and fishing with her father, "to make him happy." Her brother played sports like baseball, delivered newspapers, "and just went out"; "we didn't do things together." As a child, Eileen helped her mother with the cleaning but did very little cooking or other chores. She was unable to remember activities her mother did besides cooking and cleaning, and cleaning other people's homes for money.

Eileen's father did the repairing, had a steady job as an engineer at Bethlehem Steel, liked to work on cars, installed cement walkways, and built fishponds. She stated, "He was kind of creative. He did kind of modeling of presidents' faces with his hands with plaster-of-paris and carving. He was an intelligent, creative man for the amount of schooling he had."

AVA'S LIFESTYLE PERFORMANCE PROFILE

Ava is a 19-year-old engaged female mother who was born in Portugal, the eldest of three daughters. She and her family immigrated to the United States approximately 10 years ago. She lives with her parents who are still married. Ava was admitted to the psychiatric unit because she threatened to kill herself and stated she was very depressed. She identified her main stressor as an impaired relationship with her boyfriend who accused her of sleeping with his best friend, which she claims is not true. In addition, he threatened to terminate the relationship. She had one prior psychiatric admission to the same hospital 2 months prior because of depression and suicidal ideation. She reports that she started to have problems with depression approximately 5 years ago when she moved from New Jersey to Pennsylvania. She has a 2-year-old daughter by another man. Her diagnoses include:

Axis I: Major depression, recurrent, moderately severe

Axis II: Mixed personality disorder with histrionic, impulsive, and immature features

Axis III: Parasuicidal behavior with erythema of hand from pressing upon pins at work

Axis IV: Moderately severe: problems with boyfriend; death of grandfather

Axis V: 41.6, in the past 70.3

Ava was quite willing and positively anxious to do the interview. The occupational therapist already had a good rapport with this patient because of knowing her from a past admission. In fact, like Eileen, Ava repeatedly asked, "When are you going to interview me?" with a big smile on her face. She seemed to have no problems with the tape recorder and simply ignored it. Although she was cooperative and pleasant in the interview, the occupational therapist sensed that she was holding back information or simply glossing in an effort to be released from the unit sooner (in spite of the fact that it was clearly explained to her that this interview was confidential and had no bearing on her treatment). At the time of the interview (which occurred approximately a week after admission), Ava had experienced a lessening of symptoms and was slated for discharge the next day.

Societal Contribution

Ava appeared to enjoy and value helping others, and this was observed on the unit. She would frequently get things for elderly patients or just sit and talk to them. When asked what kinds of things she does to help other people, she states that "if it is an older person, you know I would want to make sure that she is safe... like taking care of them, make sure they have water or whatever they need." She described helping an older man in her neighborhood, giving him baths and other care-taking tasks. It is Ava's dream to become a nurse and work with older people.

Ava has worked part-time for 2 years as a folder of pleats for sofa upholstery. It is an assembly line job. Before that she worked folding shirts in a women's sportswear factory. She states that she loves her work because she likes making money and being physically active. She dislikes her boss because she states, "She is too picky, and when she gets too picky, then I start picking... behind her back." She calls in sick once or more a month and is often late when she can't get a ride. In spite of this, she believes she is a valued worker and that she does her job well, stating, "I'm one of the best folders they have." When asked what she would change about her job she replies, "Wear mini-skirts to work."

Reciprocal Interpersonal Relatedness

Ava describes having no real friends. She mentioned a former best friend whom she stopped talking to, who is also the godmother of her daughter. The physician on the team reported approximately a year ago that this best friend slept in Ava's bed with Ava's male cousin. This best friend was a virgin and left a bloodstain that Ava found. Ava warned her not to repeat this or she would tell her mother. The friend repeated this and the friendship was broken off (this information was ascertained from the physician's report, not the interview). Ava states, "I had a best friend, but my sister kind of broke-up the relationship with me and her. We just stopped seeing each other, stopped talking to each other. I don't have many friends. You know, my friend is only my kid and me, and my boyfriend." However, Ava described a neighbor, "an older lady" as the person she would call for help or talk to if she needed a confidante. "She went through the same thing, she probably could help me." She believes that she's not the type of person people take advantage of, "If they do, then they have something else coming."

Ava described a lot of conflict with her family, especially her older sister, stating, "Me and her fight a lot. We don't get along... I'm scared that I might hurt her, since I tried choking her already." "Me, I live in a house, in a house of animals... my parents they're very strict, and we just don't like being told about it, do you know what I mean? We want to do our things our way, and they don't like that, and it's hard for three girls living in one house, with three different problems, and my parents have problems of their own." In addition, she states that where she lives is too quiet and that there are no people her age to talk to. "When you have a problem, you can't go all the time to an older people."

Self-Care and Self-Maintenance

Ava lives in a large house with her parents, two sisters, fiancé, daughter, and three relatives from Portugal. It is a large house in a poor, urban area of a small city. She has lived there for 6 years and is considering moving to another small local city or to Puerto Rico. When asked about various self-maintenance tasks she described liking all of them with the exception of repairs and gardening, which she leaves to her fiancé. She especially enjoys tasks that she sees as a housewife's duties (i.e., cooking, cleaning, looking good, and grocery shopping).

Intrinsic Gratification

When asked what she likes to do for fun she replies, "Waste money. No, take care of my kid, play with her for fun. Watch TV once in a while. Listen to music (relaxation tapes)... and having sex with my man; I do everything for fun." In addition, she enjoys going to movies (especially violent, action-adventure movies) and to a local amusement park. Although she is not able to read English very well, she enjoys "reading" magazines and bride books.

As a child her favorite activity was playing nurse. She states, "Sometimes when little kids used to come over, I used to pile a bunch of papers, write their names, how sick they were, and take their temperature." She was vague when describing her sisters' activities: "We used to play with Barbies, but they stopped." Her mother was a cleaning lady and a waitress, while her father worked in construction. She stated her parents used to take her to church and to restaurants. Both of her parents are illiterate. She stated as a teenager, "I still played with Barbie. I still pretended that I was a nurse." Ava describes feeling limited by her Portuguese background, "If I was American, I think I would have more rights than an alien does. I would get picked more for a job than an alien would. Sometimes they deny you because you are an alien." When asked what kinds of things she does with her family she states, "We argue." When she is down she likes to play with her daughter. She also describes playing with her daughter as her main joyful activity.

Future

When asked what she would do if she were to win $100,000 she states, "I'd buy myself a house, a car, get whatever my daughter needs for her college, and the rest I would give it to whoever needed, poor people. Give some to the Salvation Army, the church." She believes her life will get better in the next year because she is getting married and she will "be more responsible, more independent, think about what a wife would do, not like a kid. Play with my daughter later. Take care of the house and then play with my daughter." She believes her life is good compared to a lot of women she knows.

Personal History/Culture

When asked what object she owns that tells something about her, she states her dolls, especially a Shirley Temple doll. Her favorite subjects in school were science and biology. She described difficulty in school because she didn't know English well. Also, she feels she was discriminated against because she was

Portuguese, "They used to hit me, pick on me, because I was Portuguese... No matter what kid it was, it was Portuguese, Puerto Rican, and black... those three weren't their favorites." Her least favorite subject was reading. Her chores growing up included vacuuming, cleaning, and doing the dishes, but she states, "I liked doing it." Her mother washed the clothes and cooked while her father worked and did the construction around the house.

BONNIE'S LIFESTYLE PERFORMANCE PROFILE

Bonnie is a 44-year-old white, divorced female admitted to the psychiatric unit after an overdose and suicidal intentions. According to the patient, she had been increasingly depressed. She has a history of depression during the past 4 years with one previous suicide attempt. She improved with psychotherapy and anti-depression medication, which she discontinued some time after feeling better. She indicated that lately she had been depressed and sad, and the evening before her admission she went out drinking alcohol by herself, and shortly after overdosed on coumadin. She admitted to suicidal intentions and increasing self-devaluation ideas during the last week but identifies no stressors in her life. Her job is "okay." She described her relationship with her boyfriend as fine. She described having increasingly poor self-esteem and poor sleep and appetite.

Various interdisciplinary documentation described Bonnie as having symptoms of depression starting about 4 years ago. Symptoms worsened until the point that she overdosed on her medications. She does not remember exactly the length of her treatment but indicates probably less than 1 year. She dropped treatment because she started feeling better. She denies any history of alcohol abuse and indicates she drinks only when she is very depressed. Her father committed suicide at the age of 34. She has a brother and a sister but does not know of a history of depression in them. Her diagnoses are as follows:

Axis I: Major depression, severe, recurrent, without psychotic features

Axis II: No diagnoses

Axis III: Overdose on coumadin, heart condition, two trans-ischemic attacks, scoliosis

Axis IV: Minimal

Axis V: 42/86

Bonnie was very agreeable to participating in the interview. She did not seem to mind the tape recorder. During the interview she appeared relaxed and was very talkative. She demonstrated appropriate ranges of affect and did not hesitate to answer questions.

Societal Contribution

Bonnie appears to highly value service to others and performs a number of different tasks in this area. One task is visiting her boyfriend's mother at least once a week. "I think it makes her happier... she's a little older, and this hot weather we've been having, she can't go out, she's got real bad asthma." Another task she does is to shovel the snow for her landlady. She described doing a lot for her boyfriend including his laundry, packing special lunches, and doing "odds and ends." She describes always being a caretaker for her family in Virginia. Presently, she makes up small packages for her mother containing stationery, books, and stamps. Her mother then uses the supplies to write poetry and send Bonnie her thoughts. She stated that growing up she assumed all the roles of mother for her younger sister and brother since her father committed suicide and her mother was a chronic alcoholic.

Bonnie identifies herself as a bookkeeper and has worked in various jobs including accounts payable, accounts receivable, and as a clerk in business offices and billing departments. She describes her more favorite jobs as including more contact with the general public, stating, "I think I'm a lot better off when I have a more public-oriented position than I am if I'm stuck in a little office by myself. 'Cause, I like the public real well. I like to be with people." Currently, she works full-time in an ophthalmologist's office as a bookkeeper. She describes herself as very reliable, never calling off or being late except for serious illnesses. Bonnie prides herself in her work and thinks she is both a very hard worker and a positive influence on the other staff, who she describes as negative. However, she states that although she knew "in the back of her mind" that she was a good worker, she had begun to doubt that recently. A highly complimentary phone call from her boss on the day of the interview made her feel a lot better, "I really didn't know that (I was needed) until I talked to my boss today... that made me feel good." When asked what she would like to change about her job, she replies, "I think I would make better communication for the whole business," and stressed how important good communication is in a small workplace.

Reciprocal Interpersonal Relatedness

Bonnie currently has few friends in the area, which she relates to the fact that she has relocated so much. She states that most of her friends are in Ohio and Virginia. She moved from Virginia to Ohio to be with her former husband, who lived there. She is divorced. About the divorce she states, "He was a salesman and always on business... 5 nights a week." After her divorce, she met a man who was from Pennsylvania and moved to this area because of him. "We did not work out and I didn't want to start my life over again so I stayed in Pennsylvania."

Bonnie occasionally socializes with the "girls from work" but states that she works odd hours and this prevents her from seeing them. In addition she states, "They all have a significant other or children." She mentioned spending some time with her boyfriend's sister and her landlady. Bonnie discussed one close friend from Virginia with whom she grew up. She describes her as "a good person," but seems resentful that she never visits her. "She's got the vacation, she's got the money, but she never visits me." In addition, she describes "putting a stop" to frequent visits to see her family in Virginia. She believes it is now their turn to come see her. Bonnie states that if she were afraid or needed help she would talk to her boyfriend's sister and not her close friend from home, "because she would say, 'just come home, that's why you should live here'."

Bonnie describes her relationship with her boyfriend as "having its ups and downs." They have been together for about a year and they live together. She states that he went through a bitter divorce and this makes him very cautious. She believes that they do not have a lot in common, "He likes car racing and I like going to the movies and reading." She describes one thing she does not like about him as, "He sometimes will get with the boys and sort of forget about me, like not making a phone call... I think it's rude and disrespectful and I tell him so." Bonnie describes herself as too giving sometimes. "I think sometimes I think more about the other person than about my needs."

Bonnie stated that she has decided to make more of an effort to spend more time with others: "Instead of being alone so often, I'm going to call his sisters and spend more time with another person. And he and I are going to do more things together as a couple, we discussed this the other night."

Self-Care and Self-Maintenance

Bonnie lives with her boyfriend in a spacious one-bedroom second-floor apartment with a lot of windows. The apartment is hers in that the lease is in her name and she is ultimately responsible for it. She states that it is in a quiet and safe neighborhood within walking distance to her job. She misses owning a home, but she is very happy with her current living situation. Although she is responsible for paying the bills, she claims that managing finances is her least favorite chore since she does bookkeeping all day at her job. She enjoys and is good at taking care of her clothes and laundry and maintaining her personal hygiene. She does not enjoy grocery shopping, as she states that this has become mundane. Bonnie has started to enjoy cooking more recently and actually looks forward to days when she can prepare a homemade meal for herself and her boyfriend. She is diligent about maintaining and cleaning her household, but she states this has been lacking since she has been depressed: "I do the basics... but right now, it's been kind of... I just haven't felt like doing it." She hasn't had the energy lately. "I get disgusted with myself sometimes, so then I just kind of lay it aside. I decide it's as good as it should be." In the past, Bonnie enjoyed yard work and gardening but no longer does this because she lives in an apartment.

When Bonnie was asked if she ever did not feel safe, she at first said no but changed her answer as she thought about it, "It's that I don't feel secure when I'm down... I feel unsafe, definitely. And I don't care what anyone does around me, whether it's my friends, or my boyfriend, they can't get rid of that unsafeness... I don't think anybody is going to hurt me, and I don't think as far as me hurting myself; it's just my thoughts I guess. Like, why am I down? I've got all this going on for me, why am I having these silly insecure thoughts?" As the occupational therapist discussed this feeling with her, he learned that she believed that she was afraid that something is seriously wrong with her because she feels that way. "I think that inturn makes the depression feel even worse 'cause I'm kind of beating up myself for having these thoughts."

Intrinsic Gratification

One of Bonnie's favorite activities is going to the movies, either alone or with others. She especially enjoys dramas. She also enjoys reading, "I'm a big-time reader... like a book a week... I read fiction, non-fiction, poetry, and literature." In addition, she enjoys walks, mall shopping, dining out, and going to the mountains to look at the trees when they change colors. Bonnie frequently volunteers to babysit children, "I like to do that. It makes me feel good, and it gives them a break." Bonnie also identifies cooking as a pleasurable activity. She states that most of her activities are done by herself.

As a child, Bonnie enjoyed hopscotch with her best friend but couldn't elaborate on other favorite activities. As a teenager she enjoyed going to the movies on Sunday afternoons, "'cause the movies were only 50 cents, and we were very poor, and my mother with her social security check, she would... drop us off." As a young adult she described doing volunteer work for the elderly a couple of nights a week.

When asked what she does to make herself feel good, Bonnie states that she calls her mother early in the morning (before her mother has a chance to get drunk). She takes her boyfriend's mother shopping or out to eat. Another thing that helps her feel good is clearing away clutter in her apartment and finishing paying bills and opening mail, "So when I get through all my mail and everything is taken care of, that makes me feel good."

Future

When asked what she would do if she won $100,000, she states, "I wouldn't quit my job. I'd ask if I could work part-time. I'd build myself a little home. Nothing extravagant. Get a new car, 'cause I really need a new car big-time. I would donate to charities... to children that are very disadvantaged. I would ask my family if they needed anything." She believes in a year her life will be better because she is now getting help and learning that she needs to ask for help when she's not feeling well, "I will definitely reach out." Overall, Bonnie believes her life is pretty good when compared to other people.

Personal History/Culture

When asked to describe an object that tells something about her she mentions a smiley button, which she wears almost all the time. She states, "I don't care if it's 7 o'clock in the morning, 6 o'clock, 8 o'clock, I'm smiling, and I'm just... like my boss told me (excuse my language), 'How in the hell can you be so happy at 8 o'clock in the morning?'" When asked to complete the sentence, "My family expects me to be_____" she replies, "available no matter what." When asked what she wanted to be she states, "I just want to be me... I guess I want to be respected by my family." Her favorite subjects in school were literature and poetry. Her least favorite subjects in school were geometry and chemistry.

As a child she described not doing much for fun with her family because her mother was an alcoholic. The only activities she mentioned were going to a Baptist church and going to the movies. Her brother enjoyed racing cars, and she and her mother were very artistic and both painted and wrote poetry. Bonnie had the responsibility at an early age of running the household and caring for her younger siblings. Her sister would help her as much as she could, while it was her brother's responsibility to chop wood and bring in the groceries. She stated that her father died when she was 6 or 7, and she doesn't remember much about him except that he worked in a coal mine and would bring her with him when he would play cards with the guys. Her mother worked for a short period of time in a chicken plant.

USING THE PROFILES

With information from a preliminary evaluation completed by the interdisciplinary team, the occupational therapist provides goals and intervention strategies that allow the individual with recurrent major depression to function in a less restrictive environment (outpatient counseling, psychiatric visits, support groups, etc.).

KEY POINTS

- Each Lifestyle Performance Profile is individualized.
- Within the profile, a picture or story of the person's activity emerges.
- The profile emphasizes the person's strengths and discusses needs when they impact the person's lifestyle.
- The profile forms a basis for intervention planning.
- Interpretation of the lifestyle performance and environmental profiles with accompanying information is the role of the practitioner.

REFERENCES

Estroff, S. E. (1981). *Making it crazy: An ethnography of psychiatric clients in an American community.* Berkeley, CA: University of California Press.

Fidler, G. S. (1996). Lifestyle performance: From profile to conceptual model. *Am J Occup Ther, 50,* 139-147.

Langness, L. L., & Levine, H. (Eds.). (1986). *Culture and retardation: Life histories of mildly mentally retarded persons in American society.* Norwell, MA: Kluwer Academic Publishers.

Zola, I. K. (1982). *Missing pieces: A chronicle of living with a disability.* Philadelphia: Temple University Press.

Data Interpretation and Outcome Indicators

Practicing occupational therapy using the Lifestyle Performance Model enables therapists to identify both the types and sources of data that will enable them to see the occupational therapy participant holistically. The generation of such substantive data requires a belief that it will be useful in designing intervention and that the data will be manageable. The use of the Lifestyle Performance Interview incorporates the belief that individuals are more than "information-processing machines." The interview gathers individuals' perceptions of meaning about occupations and, as such, views people as "meaning-generating beings" (Anderson & Goolishian, 1995). The environmental profile provides a perspective for both the therapist and participant to understand the context within which activities take place or are generated.

The data gathered from the interview and environmental profile provides both the therapist and the occupational therapy participant an opportunity to understand and create meaning regarding the person's lifestyle. In order to do so, the therapist needs to understand his or her role in putting together the data. As in the interview process, the therapist approaches the data from a "not knowing" stance. He or she sees the data as a way of being informed about the lifestyle of the individual. This assumes the therapist is able to maintain an attitude of "not knowing," of allowing the data to speak through the participant to inform the therapist. Using inductive reasoning, the therapist and participant create a

Lifestyle Performance Profile that represents the person's lifestyle as it exists for that moment in time. This analysis is like the analysis used in qualitative research. This narrative must represent the participant's account, not the therapist's professional account.

The narrative describes the activities within the four domains, the environment, and the value that the participant places on the needs of autonomy, individuality, affiliation, volition, consensual validation, predictability, self-efficacy, adventure, accommodation, and reflection. These needs are more fully described in Chapter 1.

To understand the participant's current quality of life from an occupational perspective, the individual with the therapist identifies the activities within each domain that most impact his or her quality of life and lists them under the relevant domain on the Quality of Life Lifestyle Review (see next page). The review is completed after the Lifestyle Performance Profile has been created. The respondent is asked to rate each activity he or she has listed regarding his or her current level of satisfaction.

The review must not be used as a way to collect normative data about quality of life or to compare individuals. Rather, it is intended to provide the participant and the therapist a way to identify how the quality of life is changing as the result of intervention. As such, it can be used to monitor intervention and as an outcome measure of intervention.

QUALITY OF LIFE LIFESTYLE REVIEW

Within each domain, list the activities that most contribute to your quality of life. For each activity, please choose the response that best describes how satisfied you are with that activity in your life. Please mark your response by circling the number. There are no right or wrong responses.

How Satisfied Are You With:

The area of reciprocal interpersonal relatedness: Activities done to sustain relationships with others.

List activities below:

	Least Satisfied						Most Satisfied
	1	2	3	4	5	6	7
	1	2	3	4	5	6	7
	1	2	3	4	5	6	7
	1	2	3	4	5	6	7
	1	2	3	4	5	6	7

The area of societal contribution: Activities done to contribute to the need fulfillment and welfare of others.

List activities below:

	Least Satisfied						Most Satisfied
	1	2	3	4	5	6	7
	1	2	3	4	5	6	7
	1	2	3	4	5	6	7
	1	2	3	4	5	6	7
	1	2	3	4	5	6	7

continued

The area of self-care and self-maintenance: Activities done to care for yourself and your personal surroundings.

List activities below:

	Least Satisfied						Most Satisfied
	1	2	3	4	5	6	7
	1	2	3	4	5	6	7
	1	2	3	4	5	6	7
	1	2	3	4	5	6	7
	1	2	3	4	5	6	7

The area of intrinsic gratification: Activities done for pleasure and enjoyment.

List activities below:

	Least Satisfied						Most Satisfied
	1	2	3	4	5	6	7
	1	2	3	4	5	6	7
	1	2	3	4	5	6	7
	1	2	3	4	5	6	7
	1	2	3	4	5	6	7

INTERPRETING THE DATA

Examination of the Lifestyle Performance Profile begins with analyzing the activities within each domain to determine the common threads. What commonalties exist in areas such as the level of creativity, structure, spontaneity, or predictability? What are the types and levels of interpersonal engagement represented within the lifestyle? How do equipment and objects typically used within activities represent the value and meaning of objects within the individual's life? Does the person prefer equipment that is power driven or hand manipulated? What types of environments are represented throughout the person's lifestyle? Are these environments supportive of or barriers to engagement? What types of activities do the environments themselves generate? Does the person have the skills and abilities to successfully participate in these activities?

The therapist also works with the participant to identify strengths and weaknesses in psychological, neurological, psychomotor, and interpersonal areas of functioning that interfere with the satisfaction equation. This may include assessments representing specific frames of reference such as biomechanical (strength), cognitive (Allen's cognitive levels), or neurodevelopmental (ability to dissociate movements). The results of these assessments are used to understand how or why the person is able to engage in activities. Restoration or establishment of function within these areas is initiated when it is deemed relevant to the participant and to engagement in desired activities.

Values and attitudes of the occupational therapy participant are relevant to the intervention process. They are most frequently accessed through questions during the interview process, inferred through observation of the individual's personal environment, or derived through conversations with significant others. They are relevant to the model because they serve as unseen guides to choices of activities and environments.

DEVELOPING AN INTERVENTION PLAN

In developing an intervention plan, the therapist works with the participant to target activities that the individual values and that address the needs of autonomy, individuality, affiliation, volition, consensual validation, predictability, self-efficacy, adventure, accommodation, and reflection. When existing activities are inadequate because the individual is no longer able to experience satisfaction, new activities may be suggested. These replacement activities may be chosen because they hold something in common with former activities. For example, the therapist working with Mr. Edmonds noticed that many of his favored activities contained rules and structure. They had components of puzzles where Mr. Edmonds "figured it out." For example, he was an avid mechanic and farmer, maintaining a budget on a limited income. Few activities were discussed that involved interpersonal relationships. He described himself as having few friends and having difficulty with "knowing how far to go and knowing what to say and not saying too much." It appears that the elements of strategy as described by Moore and Anderson (1968) were either difficult or not pleasing for him, so he chose not to do those types of activities. Further, he frequently talked about "doing it myself" or "not living by nobody's rules but mine." When the therapist examined his preferred occupations, the majority of them were solitary in nature, or if they were done around others, they did not require interaction with others in order to be successful. In choosing replacement activities for those he can no longer do because of health-related problems, the therapist would take these common elements of Mr. Edmonds' lifestyle profile into account.

When there are activities that could be personally more relevant to the individual, the therapist may suggest new activities. In reviewing the Lifestyle Performance Profile, the occupational therapist and participant may also decide to add activities to enhance a sense of harmony between the domains. A third reason for making changes in the activities composing the profile arises when the individual is unable to engage in activities generated within the environment in which he or she exists. This includes the physical and social-cultural environment.

CHOOSING ACTIVITIES

The activities are chosen based on an analysis of their characteristics. The therapist looks for new activities that contain some of the elements identified as common threads. The analysis includes the form and structure, properties, action process, and real and symbolic meaning (Fidler & Velde, 1999, pp. 54-57).

Practitioner tasks required in the process include data gathering, raising issues regarding the environmental context, clarifying the outcome of occupational therapy intervention, supporting the client through challenges, and determining occupational therapy strategies for achieving client goals. Expectations of the client in the process include determining who should be involved in the process, creating data, reflecting the data gathered, setting goals, and reviewing the process. Joint responsibilities include data interpretation through creation of a Lifestyle Performance Profile, determination of priorities, and active collaboration.

OUTCOMES

The outcome of occupational therapy practiced through the Lifestyle Performance Model is enhanced quality of life. The therapist must remember that the outcome of the model is focused on the participant's life, not the therapist's perception of the participant's life or the therapist's value system. It is possible that there is lack of agreement between the therapist and the participant regarding the quality of life. When this occurs, the therapist must question why the discrepancy occurred. Is it a difference in values between them? Is it because the participant is unaware that life could be better? Does the participant lack the skills and abilities to make changes and is therefore disempowered? Perceived quality of life is frequently evaluated against one's own peer and cohort group. Does this explain the difference in perception? The therapist faces an ethical dilemma in determining how to handle such a situation.

Finally, the Lifestyle Performance Model is in all cases a person-centered approach and may be a person-driven approach. When person-centered, the therapist and participant have a cooperative relationship. The therapist seeks participant input and ultimately integrates such input into decisions made for the intervention process.

Whenever possible, the process should be person-driven. Here, the individual assumes responsibility for decision-making with the input and consultation of the therapist. It is possible that the person perceives his or her lifestyle as adequate, while the therapist disagrees. In this case, the therapist must remember that while therapy is a socially constructed experience, it is the occupational therapy participant's truth that is being told. In the collaborative process of telling the story, the therapist may suggest alternative perspectives, but ultimately the participant's perspective must be honored and believed.

REFERENCES

Anderson, H., & Goolishian, H. (1995). The client is the expert: A not-knowing approach to therapy. In S. McNamee & K. J. Gergen (Eds.), *Therapy as social construction* (pp. 25-39). Thousand Oaks, CA: Sage.

Fidler, G. S., & Velde, B. P. (1999). *Activities: Reality and symbol.* Thorofare, NJ: SLACK Incorporated.

Moore, O. K., & Anderson, A. R. (1968). *Some principles for the design of clarifying educational environments.* Pittsburgh, PA: University of Pittsburgh, Learning Research and Development Center.

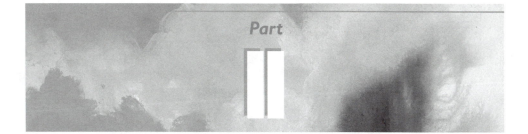

THE MODEL AT USE IN OCCUPATIONAL THERAPY PRACTICE

Part II of this book is intended to provide readers with real examples of the Lifestyle Performance Model in occupational therapy practice. The authors of Chapters 9 through 15 apply the model in their service to individuals on a regular basis. Each chapter is unique and presents the reader with a slightly different perspective of the model and its use in different systems. These chapters are not written in a rigid format, but convey to the reader the perspective of unique practitioners in their own words and style.

Presentation order of the domains is varied based upon the judgment of the authors. The domains are not viewed in a hierarchal manner, so their order of presentation is irrelevant.

Chapter 9—*Providing Services for a Child and His Family: Gregory* exemplifies the clinical reasoning processes needed to transition from the data gathered to the intervention plan established. Chapters 10 to 15 illustrate how the model tells the occupational story of persons across a wide age span residing in a variety of settings.

Chapter 16—*The Model as a Tool for Institutional Planning* illustrates how the model can be used at the organizational level. This chapter suggests changes to the institutional environment, staffing, staff training, and approach to clients that exemplify the constructs and sub-constructs of the model.

Finally, Chapter 17—*A Look to the Future* challenges readers to be critical, to contribute to scholarly debate, and to help the authors develop strategies to counteract pragmatic difficulties in implementing the model.

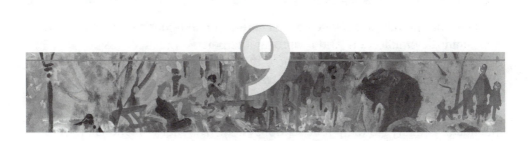

Providing Services for a Child and His Family

Gregory

Amy Gerney, MS, OTR/L and Gail S. Fidler, OTR, FAOTA

The Lifestyle Performance Model offers a refreshing new way to view individuals in school and pediatric settings. It provides a template that is helpful in setting priorities with these individuals. It provides a framework that enables the occupational therapist and client along with families and/or teachers to consider intervention strategies that are relevant to the individual and his or her environment in a context that is appropriate to his or her particular lifestyle. It is a model that is well-grounded in quality of life values and enables the occupational therapist to devise an intervention plan that specifically relates to a child's quality of life.

Educators are now discussing quality of life as it relates to their students with disabilities. They are looking far beyond literacy and handwriting legibility and are redefining outcomes for students with special needs. There seems to be recognition that there is more to educating children than just giving them "book smarts." Attention is being given to community skills, leisure skills, social skills, and related experiences. This is a welcome focus to those individuals who have long advocated such emphasis in education.

The Lifestyle Performance Model offers an exciting new look at individuals with developmental disabilities through their life span as well as those found in pediatric settings, including the public schools (inclusive of high school). It is congruent with the emphasis that educators are currently placing on quality of life. The model clearly articulates quality of life as related to harmony among four domains that pertain to activities of self-care/self-maintenance, societal contributions, intrinsic gratification, and reciprocal interpersonal relatedness.

The following material describes how this model was applied in the case of a 5-year-old child with Down syndrome who was transitioning from an early intervention program into an inclusive kindergarten at a public school.

What follows is a document that was used as a way of introducing such an individual—Gregory—to the public school system. The mother, who is an occupational therapist, wished for her child to be viewed not as a laundry list of deficits, as is traditional, but as a human being with strengths and needs. She wanted for her son's new "team" to understand him in a novel way—from a perspective of Gregory's lifestyle, rich with charm and laughter along with the challenges that the Down syndrome posed. What follows is a Lifestyle Performance Profile of Gregory written specifically for a team of educators. It was presented at the transition meeting from early intervention services to kindergarten.

INFORMATION PRESENTED TO THE INDIVIDUAL EDUCATION PLAN TEAM

The Lifestyle Performance Model is based on the belief that in order to "sustain health and enable life satisfaction" there needs to be a sense of harmony among four activity domains. In looking at Gregory, we would like to see some sense of autonomy in his ability to care for his personal needs, not only for himself but also for his work, living space, and surroundings. We also would like to foster his ability to contribute to the well-being of others, develop connectedness to other individuals, and grow and develop skills and interests that will enable him to have fun.

LIFESTYLE PERFORMANCE PROFILE: G.G. 3/99

Self-Care and Self-Maintenance

Gregory demonstrates an interest in his personal appearance. He will stand in front of a mirror with prompts and comb his hair, "fix his shirt," and wipe a missed spot of food from his chin. He brushes his teeth with "set-up" and will wash his hands if the water is regulated. In the bathtub, he washes himself with verbal prompts. Gregory is able to put on his shoes but not tie them. He can take off his coat and put it back on with "set-up." He can manage the zipper of his coat once it is started. Gregory will make his bed with help and picks up his own toys with verbal prompts. He clears his own place setting and wipes up his own spills, picks up his own clothes and puts them with the dirty clothes. He likes to help vacuum and dust, and makes crude attempts to wash windows. He role-plays many domestic chores. Gregory can feed himself once the containers are opened and the food is cut. He is able to drink from a glass when it is partially filled. He can be very sloppy at times with consistencies such as pudding, ice cream, yogurt, etc. He joins his family for meal times and conducts himself appropriately. He eats out frequently in restaurants with his family.

Areas of Need With Regard to Self-Care and Self-Maintenance

Gregory needs to learn to toilet himself. We are hopeful that he will be independent with this skill with reminders once the academic year begins this fall. He also needs to internalize picking up after himself. For many of these skills that are emerging, he does quite well but does not initiate and currently needs a lot of cues and structure. He has the idea and the desire to perform tasks independently but needs further refinement of the skills to complete them successfully.

Societal Contribution

Gregory helps his brothers with their chores of emptying the dishwasher, taking out trash, etc. He will set the table with cues, carry out a bag of trash (paper) to the garage, and put clothes into the dryer. He does a lot of modeling play where he serves "play meals" and does chores. Gregory also likes to make things for others. Often, when faced with a task that is frustrating, his teacher/therapist will prompt him by saying, "Make this for daddy," or "We'll hang this in daddy's office when we're done." He was very interested in giving valentines and likes to pass things out.

Gregory also knows all of the delivery service drivers who frequently come to his home for his father's home office. He greets them at the front door (with supervision), picks up or delivers the package, and takes it to his dad's desk. He also takes pride in delivering his dad's business correspondence to a mailbox.

Areas of Need With Regard to Societal Contribution

Gregory will readily engage in an activity when he feels like he is helping. This is one area that he consistently initiates. If he sees his mom doing laundry, he will approach and point to himself and say "elp" to say "I want to help." He needs to have practice in order to further refine these skills, along with added responsibility as he gains independence. Gregory should soon be able to handle small chores of his own.

Reciprocal Interpersonal Relatedness

If something gets a laugh, Gregory will repeat it. He enjoys "performing" when others respond positively toward him. Of course, this isn't always positive and other children have been found to reinforce a negative behavior by laughing.

Gregory is easily led astray by others, and in public situations approaches strangers and at times says "up" to request a stranger to hold him. He easily relates to new caretakers, such as in the church nursery where the caretaker changes from week to week. He readily separates from his parents.

Gregory easily becomes frustrated in a play situation when someone takes a toy from him. In this situation, he will hit, say "jerk," and try to grab the toy. Those who are familiar with Gregory (e.g., his brothers) know not to frustrate him in this way, but in new situations the language barrier makes such encounters frustrating for Gregory. More recently, he has begun to come and get mom or dad and make attempts to explain his frustration by yelling, pointing, and motioning to "come here."

Gregory has developed close relationships with his two older brothers, ages 11 and 7, as well as his parents. He demonstrates a great deal of affection, gives great hugs, and shows concern when another person is crying. He also shows interest in those who are hurt, often pointing out pictures in books of kids in a cast. At the nursing home where he visits, he shows concern for those in a wheelchair by signing the sign for "hurt." Many an intervention session has been interrupted by his preoccupation with a "boo-boo" on a therapist's/teacher's hand. He is quick to point out such anomalies.

Gregory's preschool teacher has shared that there have been a lot of really nice interactions with the other 12 children at his school. He reportedly plays well with others (3- to 5-year-olds) in a playground situation with appropriate interactions, taking turns and sharing. He readily nuzzles up with other children to look at a book together.

In family situations, he is developing some nice close ties that are expanding into the extended family with an interest in his cousin Ashley. When he is proud of something, he makes the sign for the phone and says "Ash."

Gregory has an exceptional attachment to his dog Dilbert or "Bert." Every morning he goes to the front door and yells "Dilbert," whistles, and slaps his thigh to call the dog back into the house. He very clearly articulates "stay" when he wants Dilbert to hang out in his room. At bedtime, Gregory says, "Mom out, Dilbert stay," which to date is his longest chain of words. He seeks out Dilbert when he is hurting or being disciplined.

Areas of Need With Regard to Reciprocal Interpersonal Relatedness

Gregory appears most limited by his communication deficits. He is developing some nice relationships in contexts where his deficits are accepted. His adjustment to the preschool situation with regard to the other children has been for the most part positive, however by no means normal. His involvement with the other children in the neighborhood is limited to children gathering at his house. He isn't allowed to go to other houses because of his limited toileting skills and his impulsivity that manifests itself in his tendency to run away. It is important to note that one of his resources is that he is welcome in other homes with the neighborhood children.

Intrinsic Gratification

Gregory loves books. A major part of his solitary play is spent looking at picture books. He will sit and listen to someone reading to him for up to 5 minutes, 10 to 12 books at a time. Gregory also likes matchbox cars, trains, and action figures, often lining up these items. His favorite movie is *Home Alone*, which he requests by making the famous yell with his hands on his cheeks. He loves being outside doing almost anything—digging in the garden or sandbox, swinging or walking (he especially likes walks in the woods). He enjoys swimming and looks forward to frequent business trips with his father when he can swim in hotel pools. He has just learned to swim on his own with water wings. He likes *Arthur, Madeline* (books and TV), music (drums), and ice cream.

Gregory is often included in backyard ball games with his older brothers—soccer, football, baseball, and basketball. (He is often excluded from backyard games when the neighborhood kids are involved, but this is primarily due to his skill level.) He has a great sense of humor and likes to be on the go. He initiates play activity and is never found just sitting around.

Gregory enjoys a wide array of activities but isn't really proficient in any one area. His gross motor deficits do limit his ability to participate in the neighborhood ball games, which are a major component of his two older brothers' leisure life. His older brothers are very athletic, so Gregory gets many opportunities for exposure to sporting events, however he has gross motor and cognitive delays which preclude participation at his age-appropriate level. For example, he will not be able to participate in micro-soccer, a chronologically appropriate activity, this year.

Areas of Need With Regard to Intrinsic Gratification

As Gregory grows, we would expect him to continue to explore and refine his interests. We would then expect him to develop more proficiency in a more selective array of leisure pursuits. We would also expect him to develop some skills in areas that will be with him throughout his life. These may include activities that require less physical agility and cognitive skill (strategy) such as swimming, bowling, and hiking, or activities that allow him to be a participant observer such as going to games, sports meets, theater, or concerts.

Skill Strengths and Limitations

Gregory's limitations are well-documented by the professionals who have had the pleasure of working with him over the past 5 years and include speech therapy, occupational therapy, and early intervention teaching. These limitations include cognitive, physical, social, communication, and adaptive skills.

In addition to these limitations, Gregory also runs away. He demonstrates this impulsive behavior unpredictably, which has limited his participation in a wide array of activities and events. He will find an opening in any given situation and run as fast as he can. He has found his way through an outdoor playground fence at a local day care, which precipitated his expulsion. He has "taken off" at home, usually running full speed away from the house. At home, possible exits are limited by an alarm on the lower-level door. Gregory isn't allowed to go to the neighbors' homes with his brothers, limiting social contact with other kids because of this behavior. Very often his parents choose to put Gregory in a stroller in such settings as a crowded mall, airport, or recently at Disney World to ensure his safety. At his brothers' sporting events, Gregory plays on a blanket, which provides clear boundaries.

Gregory has a fairly low frustration tolerance and will often "turn off" a therapist/teacher by disengaging from an activity if it proves uninteresting or too challenging. Strategies that have helped Gregory be successful in these situations have included, "Help me finish this Gregory," "Help me clean up so we can get another toy," "Finish this for Daddy and we'll hang it up," and/or "Do one more and we'll put it away." His strengths include his good-natured personality (he can be a charmer) and his willingness to explore his environment.

Resources

Gregory has been blessed with a wide array of professionals who have worked diligently with him over the years. He has a primary caretaker who is well-educated (with a teaching certificate) and values learning and independence. Gregory has two older brothers who are independent, active, intelligent, and self-driven. These brothers include Gregory in their daily activities and are usually very tolerant of his behavior. Gregory lives in a neighborhood of children who have been very accepting and welcoming. As a group, these kids are physically very active.

Gregory's extended family has been very supportive, offering respite for the immediate family. A teacher who has extensive experience as an early intervention teacher and knows sign language teaches his preschool.

Gregory has the opportunity to experience many activities. He goes to sporting events, travels (he's been to Costa Rica, Disney World, and camping in Maine), and participates in the community (he eats out often, goes to movies, goes to preschool two times a week, and is involved in Kindermusik).

Learning Style

Gregory imitates other people's behaviors. He will often perform a task more readily if it is demonstrated or if one works alongside of him. He likes to "do" and is active. He enjoys books and will often respond better to "show me the yellow truck" within the context of a book or within an array of matchbox trucks rather than a more sterile situation of a standardized test.

He responds well to time-out, however this requires one-on-one attention, as he will not stay in the time-out chair without supervision. He also responds well to 1-2-3 count: "Gregory, do you need help? I'm going to count to 3 and then I'm going to help." He also responds to bribes: "If you eat this you'll get ice cream" or "If you pick up your toys we'll go outside."

Gregory also needs a great deal of structure and boundaries. He does better if his chair is "wedged in" to limit a quick escape. He is more successful in a group of children sitting on the floor listening to a story if he is seated in the center of the children rather than on the outer border. He also does well when he is asked to sit on a piece of carpet along with the other children for story time. For any given task, he does better with stimuli on his workspace limited to just what he needs at that particular moment. For example, if the task involves cutting and pasting, presenting the scissors then putting them away, and then presenting the paste enables Gregory to handle the task more successfully.

IMPLEMENTATION OF THE MODEL

This Lifestyle Performance Profile paints a picture of Gregory's lifestyle. The information can be gathered through interview, record review, and observation. Open-ended questions such as, "Tell me about a typical day in your household or a typical day for Gregory in school," "Tell me about the type of activities that Gregory enjoys," "Tell me about the toys that he seems to gravitate toward," "How does he spend his time?" "Describe how he and his brothers help out around the house or how he and the other students help out in the classroom." "Who does Gregory play with and how do they play?" "Describe Gregory's morning routine or describe his lunchtime routine." Questions directed at gaining a perspective of how Gregory functions in each of the domains will yield the Lifestyle Performance Profile.

The profile will depict who Gregory is—what his activity patterns and interests are. It will also describe the demands of the environment in which he lives. Once this profile has been completed, the next step in utilizing this model would be to consider whether there is a sense of autonomy in each of the four domains and also whether there is harmony among the domains. In looking at each domain, the following areas of limitation as well as secondary dysfunction can be identified:

❧ **Self-Care and Self-Maintenance:**

Gregory needs to learn to toilet and pick up after himself.

❧ **Societal Contribution:**

Gregory needs to perform simple chores.

❧ **Reciprocal Interpersonal Relatedness:**

Gregory needs to demonstrate functional communication.

❧ **Intrinsic Gratification:**

Gregory needs to develop autonomy with enjoying books.

Gregory needs to develop skills to participate in organized sports (i.e., micro-soccer).

Gregory participates in a narrow array of interests.

❧ **Secondary Dysfunction:**

> Gregory demonstrates impulsive behavior (exiting behavior) that poses a safety concern.

When you consider the harmony among the domains in regard to Gregory, you might conclude that his areas of deficit are more pronounced in self-care and self-maintenance as well as reciprocal interpersonal relatedness. Although he does not contribute much to the welfare of others, it is important to consider his age and culture. He does not demonstrate autonomy, and he has a rather narrow array of play behavior in comparison to other children his age; but he does nonetheless play and he is happy when he plays. When you draw these types of conclusions, you hone in on those areas of Gregory's lifestyle that are not in harmony with the demands of his environment (e.g., it is important to understand that other kids his age in his community are playing micro-soccer, that his two older brothers are playing soccer, and his father is sports-minded). You place your decisions and draw your conclusions based on Gregory's lifestyle, which is a product of who he is, what he does, where he lives, with whom he lives, how he spends his time, and what demands are placed on him. Only in this context can you determine where his deficits lie and where to focus your plan of intervention.

Goals for Gregory

Once these areas of limitation have been identified, you could easily turn these into long-term goals as follows:

❧ **Self-Care and Self-Maintenance:**

> Gregory will demonstrate independence in toileting.
>
> Gregory will demonstrate independence in picking up after himself.

❧ **Societal Contribution:**

> Gregory will demonstrate independence in performing simple chores.

❧ **Reciprocal Interpersonal Relatedness:**

> Gregory will demonstrate functional communication.
>
> Gregory will demonstrate sensitivity in regard to other people's concerns.

❧ **Intrinsic Gratification:**

> Gregory will enjoy books independently.
>
> Gregory will successfully participate in backyard sports.
>
> Gregory will successfully participate in three new pleasurable activities.

You could also include a goal that addresses the secondary dysfunction of his bolting behavior as such:

> Gregory will demonstrate control of his impulses.

Performance Components

The next step in implementing the model would be to determine what per-formance components affect those domains in which autonomy is a problem. Instead of filling out a protocol assessment for a child with Down syndrome, the therapist should ask, "What is getting in the way of autonomy in each domain and harmony among the domains?" This is not a minor detail; in fact, it is a hallmark of implementing the Lifestyle Performance Model. Once the client (or parent) and therapist have painted the profile, a decision is made as to what components are negatively impacting one or more domains. The occupational therapist's judg-ment is required to determine which performance components to further assess. One should only assess those performance components that the occupational therapist has determined are impeding his sense of autonomy.

Using Frames of Reference

The occupational therapist could choose to assess Gregory's motor perform-ance. Certainly he or she might look at Gregory's motor performance using a neuro-developmental treatment (NDT) approach. This would look at hypotonicity and how the tone influences his performance with his motor skills. It would also yield a hand function assessment and his readiness to participate in fine motor activities, like turning the pages in a book, in addition to the gross motor skills, like his backyard sports. Looking at Gregory from a sensory integration (SI) per-spective would yield a wealth of information about how he is processing stimuli from his environment. For example, a therapist would want to observe Gregory, perhaps even ask staff to keep a log of the events that lead up to his "exits." What makes him pick up and walk off? Why does he crawl under the table when given certain tasks? One could take a closer look at the environment: What is the devel-opmental level of the material being presented? What else is going on in the room? Can Gregory see what's being presented? Is a vision screening warranted?

Any frame of reference can be implemented using the Lifestyle Performance Model. You can use NDT, SI, Brunnstrom, or Rood for example. The model does not restrict the use of evaluation tools or intervention strategies. Any assessment tool could be used within the larger framework of the model so long as it aids the therapist in further honing in on why there isn't autonomy. What is getting in the way of autonomy within each domain? The model simply provides the big pic-ture; it offers the framework of a person's lifestyle from which the assessment becomes further and further refined.

Summary of Assessment Information

Once the assessment has been completed, it could be summarized as follows:

Level of performance: From the psychologist's report, Gregory has been found to be mildly mentally retarded. He has an attention span of 45 seconds for tasks that he finds frustrating and can attend to a book being read to him for 5 minutes in the classroom. He appears to be easily distracted by the classroom environment and either crawls under the table or runs out of the room an average of five times per day. His classroom teacher and teacher's aide report that he does this during morning discussions about the weather and when practicing writing his name. Attempts at correcting his behavior have to date focused on reacting to the behavior with time-outs and removal of privileges. A visual screening reveals that Gregory makes one or two attempts at a fine motor task and then appears to give up in frustration. He also holds his head exceptionally close to the paper when given a paper/pencil task.

Gregory continues to wear a diaper but does indicate that he wants to be changed. Frequent attempts to toilet train have proven unsuccessful. Gregory demonstrates reduced tone. He has difficulty maintaining the extended position while in prone on the scooter board. He is unable to sustain grasp on a trapeze using both hands. He is unable to jump in place or stand on one foot. He utilizes an immature grasp for holding a pencil or paintbrush, as he is unable to demonstrate a tripod grasp.

Gregory uses approximately 30 signs, some of which have been adapted because of his immature hand development. He is able to clearly articulate approximately 10 words: stop, no, more, me, Bert and Dilbert (his dog), jerk, mom, out, and stay.

From this summary of Gregory's level of performance, the therapist should have a clearer understanding of what performance components are negatively impacting autonomy in the domains—the toileting, doing chores, functional communication, reading books, etc. These performance components are *related* to Gregory's world. It should be noted that the assessment and goals related here are by no means complete, but rather are offered as abbreviated examples of how to apply the model. One could organize the short-term goals from the assessment of the performance components as follows.

Short-Term Goals

❦ Self-Care and Self-Maintenance

Gregory will demonstrate independence in toileting.

- Gregory will demonstrate pulling his pants up and down.
- Gregory will participate in a formal toileting program based on behavioral techniques.

Gregory will demonstrate independence in picking up after himself.

- Gregory will have the opportunity to model his behavior after other children in his class, using verbal prompts and hand-over-hand to clean his workspace.

❧ Societal Contribution

Gregory will demonstrate independence in performing simple chores.

- Gregory will learn one new chore a month using chaining techniques.
- Gregory's family and aide will demonstrate a good understanding of chaining techniques in order to teach Gregory new skills.
- Gregory will pass out cups for snack time with supervision.

❧ Reciprocal Interpersonal Relatedness

Gregory will demonstrate functional communication.

- Gregory will demonstrate proficiency with and incorporate toys such as the kazoo and toy horn into his daily play routine in order to facilitate normalization of tone needed for talking (oral motor control and diaphragmatic breathing).
- Gregory will develop new hand signs in conjunction with the speech therapist that will be adapted to his (hand) developmental level.

Gregory will demonstrate sensitivity in regard to other people's concerns.

- Gregory will demonstrate a beginning awareness of how his behavior affects other people.

❧ Intrinsic Gratification

Gregory will enjoy books independently.

- Gregory will concentrate on a picture book independently for 3 minutes in the classroom.
- Gregory will demonstrate independence in operating an age-appropriate tape player to activate a talking book.
- Gregory will demonstrate independence manipulating books with sound effects on a panel down the right-hand side of the book.
- Gregory will demonstrate proficient hand skills for turning pages independently.

Gregory will successfully participate in backyard sports.

- Gregory will demonstrate reciprocal movements and muscle tone sufficient for kicking a soccer ball, catching and throwing a football, and shooting a child-sized basketball into a low basket.
- Gregory will demonstrate proficiency at taking turns.

Gregory will successfully participate in three new pleasurable activities.

- Gregory will demonstrate proficiency in painting with watercolors by structuring steps of the task and building the handle of the brush for a functional grasp.
- Gregory will demonstrate proficiency jumping on a small trampoline.
- Gregory will demonstrate proficiency in bumper bowling with some assistance.

The short-term goals to address the secondary dysfunction could be written as follows:

Gregory will demonstrate control of his impulses. Exiting behavior will be extinguished.

• Gregory will develop an attention span of 10 minutes.

• Gregory will communicate his frustration and will vocalize the word "stop" when he wants to quit a task.

• Gregory will be referred for a visual assessment.

From these goals, a plan of intervention should emerge that carries with it relevance to Gregory's lifestyle. The plan of intervention should have a direct impact on improving the quality of life for Gregory. It should include activities that help him develop a sense of autonomy in each of the domains.

Gregory's actual intervention strategies included activities that focused on pre-writing skills, stimuli (such as a weighted vest) that would give him proprioceptive input to control behavior (the running away), a limitation of stimuli (extraneous objects were removed from his work space), as well as other activities. In addition, attention was given to controlling his environment with strategies such as placing Gregory in the middle of a group of children when sitting on the floor for story time, thus making an untimely exit difficult. The therapist also guided the use of small "jobs" such as holding a basket of felt weather signs (clouds, lightening bolts, and the sun) for the teacher when concepts such as the current weather, which were too high-level for Gregory, were discussed and illustrated using a felt board. This chore helped diminish his exiting behavior. Cues such as "follow John's red shirt" and placing him in the middle enabled Gregory to develop independence in walking in lines in the school hallway.

The Lifestyle Performance Model addresses the environment as it relates to the four domains. A lot of attention was also given at home to alter Gregory's environment so that he could be successful in each of these domains. In regard to *self-care and self-maintenance*, attention to detail such as juice boxes on the door of the refrigerator within easy reach, healthy snacks in the lower kitchen drawers, elastic waistbands on his pants, and a stool at the sink made independence easy for Gregory. Drawers in his bedroom were organized into single-use drawers so that each drawer held only one type of clothing (one drawer for shorts, one for pajamas, one for long pants) so that he was able to take a clothes basket full of his clean clothes and successfully put them away. In consideration of *societal contribution*, the silverware drawer was organized similarly so that he developed competence emptying the dishwasher of silverware. Music from Kindermusik was used regularly in the car for stimulation and for the benefit of repetition to the routines, such as the hand motions for "The Wheels on the Bus" in order to foster *intrinsic gratification*. Gregory developed a sense of autonomy operating his tape recorder that played books on tapes. Gregory regularly played soccer in his backyard. Attending birthday parties facilitated his *reciprocal interpersonal relationships*.

Hosting a small party for Gregory encouraged friendships. Students from his class came to Gregory's house to play, and Gregory was encouraged to talk on the phone with his father regularly. In order to address his *secondary dysfunction*, alarms were placed on the outside doors in order to monitor his running away behavior and were removed after shaping his behavior with time-outs was successful in helping him control his impulses. All of these activities in the home incorporated the four domains and set the stage for a healthy lifestyle.

The word *independence* stated in the goals was chosen deliberately because it was felt that independence was indeed realistic, however it should be noted that the word *autonomously* could have just as easily been used if more appropriate. For example, for a child with cerebral palsy who is physically unable and will continue to be unable to write his name, a goal such as "Mark will demonstrate autonomy in writing his name" would be appropriate. The therapist would then facilitate this sense of autonomy by modifying the task and incorporating use of a name stamp or the computer. A housewife with multiple sclerosis may not have the physical capacity or desire to be independent in cleaning her house, but she certainly can develop a sense of autonomy by making the decisions about *who* cleans her house, *how* her house is cleaned, *when* her house is cleaned, and even *if* her house is cleaned. A goal that states, "Mary will demonstrate a sense of autonomy in her housekeeping responsibilities" carries with it a much different meaning than "Mary will demonstrate independence with her housekeeping responsibilities." As Gregory gets older and his ability to acquire new skills begins to level off, decisions will need to be made to foster autonomy rather that independence. For example, a goal such as "Gregory will demonstrate independence in driving" may not be realistic, but certainly "Gregory will demonstrate a sense of autonomy with mobility throughout his community" would be reasonable.

It is also important to note that one of the hallmarks of the Lifestyle Performance Model is the identification of an individual's strengths. This is just as important to the intervention process as the identification of weaknesses or deficits. The model does not advocate the amelioration of deficits, but rather finding autonomy and balance. This can be done sometimes just as easily by finding ways to capitalize on an individual's strengths. Finding strengths and reinforcing those strengths can be just as powerful to the intervention process—to improving an individual's quality of life—as "fixing" a deficit. Gregory has a gift. He is a charmer. He readily engages with people, and most people who interact with him enjoy him. It is important to provide opportunities for Gregory to further develop and refine these social skills even to the extent that they may be above average for his age. A goal to demonstrate sensitivity in regard to other people's concerns, to demonstrate a beginning awareness of how his behavior affects other people, is certainly reasonable for Gregory. It capitalizes on a skill to further develop in an area that Gregory shows some promise and potential. Providing feedback to Gregory such as, "You took that toy, Tom is mad," "Nice sharing, Katie is smiling," "Great picture, Dad will be happy," can be used to foster such awareness. This consensual validation is also one of the characteristics of the Lifestyle Performance Model.

The point of all these intervention strategies is that they relate to the enhancement of Gregory's lifestyle–to his quality of life–the essence of the Lifestyle Performance Model.

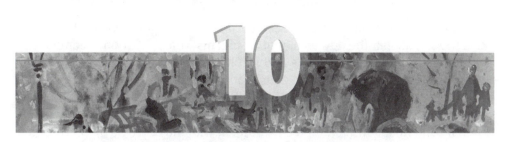

Providing Services for Elders in a Community Setting

Mrs. Scotland

Beth P. Velde, PhD, OTR/L; Peggy P. Wittman, EdD, OTR/L, FAOTA; Amy Flowers, OTR/L; Matt Stinson, OTR/L; and Peter Balent, OTR/L

Providing occupational therapy services in a system of health care built by a community requires the adaptability and flexibility to include community members as an intrinsic part of the health service team. It also requires a model of occupational therapy practice that is able to address a variety of systems whose behavior and interaction with each other can best be described as chaotic. The Lifestyle Performance Model was chosen to provide a framework for the provision of occupational therapy services in Tillery, NC. The Tillery experience included gathering data about populations and individual clients, designing intervention for individual clients, evaluating services, and conducting a qualitative research study within the parameters directed by the community of Tillery.

THE LIFESTYLE PERFORMANCE MODEL AND OCCUPATIONAL THERAPY

Faculty and students from the Occupational Therapy Department at East Carolina University have been involved with Tillery citizens through a Learn and Serve American Grant for the past 4 years. Originally funded to gather data regarding the health needs of Tillery citizens, the project continued by providing community and home-based occupational therapy using an interdisciplinary model. Faculty and students from the physical therapy department worked directly with occupational therapy faculty and students in teams to offer comprehensive services. In addition, students and faculty from the departments of exercise physiology, recreation, and health education were part of the Tillery experience.

Occupational therapy faculty believed that the Lifestyle Performance Model was the best model of practice available for use in Tillery because of its emphasis on the inter-relationship of the environment with the domains of intrinsic gratification, social contribution, self-care and self-maintenance, and interpersonal relatedness. It provided a theoretical and practical way to assess strengths, limitations, and needs of individual clients for planning intervention. In addition, the use of interview methodology as a basis for data collection provided the occupational therapists with a personal and in-depth view of the meaning of occupations to the Tillery residents as well as established a collaborative working relationship. Based on results of each individual's Lifestyle Performance Profile, frames of reference were selected for use including biomechanical, acquisitional, and cognitive.

THE TILLERY COMMUNITY

Forty acres and a mule. This was the promise given to African-American men who agreed to homestead land in rural, eastern North Carolina as part of a "resettlement community." These communities, established in 1935 by Franklin D. Roosevelt's New Deal plans, were intended to deal with "the care of needy persons in rural areas [whose] problem[s are] quite distinct and apart from that of the industrial unemployed. Their security must be identified with agriculture. They must be placed in positions of self-support" (Foreman, 1934). One of the homesteads emerging from this program was the small North Carolina community known as Tillery. Today, Tillery has few young families, and the once profitable farming community has been reduced to struggling peanut and cotton farms that dot the landscape. The economic base has severely declined, and most opportunities for jobs must be explored outside the Tillery community. The demographic characteristics of Tillery's 3,000 citizens include: 98% African-Americans, 75% over the age of 65, and 90% below the federal poverty level. One Tillery resident writes, "Tillery typifies the many rural crossroads communities in eastern North Carolina in which poverty, high unemployment, persistent racial inequities, and isolation create a very visible atmosphere of apathy and hopelessness" (Cotton, 1993, p. 2485).

Yet, antithetically, in many ways Tillery serves as a model of community involvement, change, and hope for the future. The active Concerned Citizens of Tillery organization was born 20 years ago to serve as a catalyst for not only survival, but also growth and development of the community and its citizens (20th Anniversary Celebration of the Concerned Citizens of Tillery, 1998). Today, this organization continues to be a forerunner in its efforts to provide model programs for effective land use, support to citizens of all ages, and local health care.

The strength of the Tillery community may well lie in the continuity of its occupations and availability of life roles to its residents. Occupational science defines occupations as "chunks of activity that are culturally and personally meaningful, such as dining, reading, or fishing" (Jackson, Carlson, Mandel, Zemke, & Clark, 1998, p. 327). These occupations are identified and articulated through the culture and are necessary in order to fulfill role obligations that contribute to the lifestyle of their performers. Given Tillery's history as a resettlement community, many of its citizens were engaged in farming, child-rearing, and homemaking during their childhood and adult years. As technology replaces small family farming and the citizens have reached old age and retirement, it is less clear what occupations and life roles are meaningful and help to sustain the lifestyles of Tillery residents in healthy and satisfying ways.

INDIVIDUAL ASSESSMENT AND INTERVENTION

From the perspective of occupational therapy intervention, the Lifestyle Performance Model offered the occupational therapists and occupational therapy students a frame to view the lifestyles of Tillery residents as well as a method for addressing strengths and weaknesses and for creating a plan to address them. To describe this process, we will focus on one of the residents who was a client of the interdisciplinary teams.

Mrs. Scotland is an 88-year-old widow who lives in a one-story brick home with her son. The house is located on a road with three other houses but no close neighbors. Next to the house is an old barn that is currently not being used. Across the front of her home is a concrete porch that is large enough to hold a chair where the occupant has a clear view of the road and the front yard.

Entering the front door into the living room there is a couch, non-cable television, and Mrs. Scotland's chair where she sits most of the time. She has all her bills, magazines, letters, and anything else she needs next to her chair on a small table. Her walls are covered with pictures of her family. One picture stands out—it is an 8 x 10 black & white of Mrs. Scotland with her husband taken many years ago.

In her kitchen there is a gas stove, refrigerator, and a kitchen table. Her cupboards are clearly accessible. Off the kitchen are storage and laundry rooms. Exiting the back door, there are four brick steps without a railing. There is a clothes line where she hangs her laundry and a nice size backyard with a propane tank used to fuel the stove and furnace. Adjacent to the yard is a peanut and soybean field.

Mrs. Scotland's home has two bedrooms—one for herself and one for her son. Her bedroom has a bath immediately adjacent to it. Her dresser is filled with personal items and her walls include religious icons and church service awards.

Smoke detectors are present in the home but are not working. The tub in Mrs. Scotland's bath has a low side, but she expresses some concerns for her safety when entering and exiting.

Self-Care and Self-Maintenance

Current Status and Strengths

Mrs. Scotland wakes at 5 a.m. By 6 a.m., she is ready to get out of bed to turn the heat on, "wash up," and brush her teeth. She takes a bath at night and "sprinkles" in the morning. She makes her breakfast at about 7:30 a.m. She enjoys bacon, grits, toast, and orange juice. Every other day she has croaker or pan trout. Because she has such a substantial breakfast, she eats a small lunch. Following breakfast, she checks the mail and sits down in her chair to read it. Supper is at 4 p.m.; on Thursday, Meals on Wheels provides her food. An aide has been coming in a few days a week to assist her with cooking, washing dishes, cleaning, and checking the mail.

She likes to get dressed up for church. Her hair care includes rolling her hair. She also likes to use cream on her skin everyday. She has always been an active person and stills walks and attends Friday exercise classes when they are offered.

Her yard is kept clean by cutting the grass and pulling the weeds. Flowerbeds adorn the front yard in front of the porch and under a large tree. Doing yard work has been more difficult lately and a friend comes by to assist. She does not drive, so she is dependent on her aide or her son to take her shopping for food or clothing. She manages her own money, using the ATM and food stamps to acquire items. She uses a budget to maintain her finances.

Values and Attitudes

Mrs. Scotland values doing her own self-care and self-maintenance. For example, she likes to wash her own dishes because then she knows they are clean. She follows her mother's habit of keeping her house "straight." As she says, "You could practically eat off my mama's floor." She loves eating healthy and particularly enjoys fresh fish.

Needs

Her biggest complaint is her "stiff back and sore knees," caused by arthritis and the aging process. This has decreased her gait, especially outdoors. She has some balance problems, perhaps associated with the pain and stiffness in her lower extremities. Because she does not drive, it is difficult for her to acquire self-care items, food, and health needs. Friday exercise classes will end in November, limiting her supervised exercise program.

Intrinsic Gratification

Current Status and Strengths

In the past, Mrs. Scotland was an avid seamstress, making her own clothes and the clothing for others. Her favorite past-time is fishing. She never feels stressed when sewing or fishing because she says, "I feel good at sewing and fishing." Quilting is an activity she does just for herself. These three activities are seldom part of her repertoire at this time. She enjoys spending time with others, especially at church or at the community center, where she "sings, we take exercise together, and all that stuff like that. I like to be with people, you can talk, I love that." When there is nothing else to do, she watches television, especially "kicker man" (Chuck Norris starring in *Walker: Texas Ranger*). She uses a cane when walking outside her home.

Values and Attitudes

Mrs. Scotland values the natural environment and her activities support that. Her yard is filled with flowers and she is conscious of how the environment is impacted by humans—especially the local hog farmers. Mrs. Scotland, as part of the Concerned Citizens of Tillery, has been actively opposing the use of the land around Tillery for corporate hog farms because of the potential damage to the residents' well water caused by hog waste and the negative impact on air quality.

Needs

Because her sewing machine is broken, she is unable to maintain her role as seamstress and quilter. She expresses reluctance at asking others for rides to church and the community center. Further, her arthritis makes it difficult to garden and to get to the river to go fishing. Her left wrist is swollen, probably related to a history of wrist fracture and complicated by arthritis. Her right ankle points outward as a result of an ankle fracture. These former injuries constrain her ability to fulfill her desire to be outdoors and to quilt.

Reciprocal Interpersonal Relatedness

Current Status and Strengths

Mrs. Scotland speaks strongly about her relationship with the Lord and feels she "is what she is because of Him." Many of her social connections exist through the church where she is a deaconess. Because her family lives a fair distance away, she does not see them much; however, she speaks with them frequently on the phone. She has one long-time friend to whom she is still close. "She was a friend, anything I need, all I had to do was just let her know." They currently see each other only at the community center on Tuesdays.

Values and Attitudes

Mrs. Scotland's strong belief in God shapes the majority of her actions. She believes in treating others the way she would want to be treated.

Needs

It is difficult for Mrs. Scotland to get to church activities to the extent she would like because of transportation problems and her arthritis. Her face-to-face social opportunities elsewhere in the community are also constrained by lack of transportation.

Societal Contribution

Current Status and Strengths

Of the four domains, this area contains numerous past and current activities. Mrs. Scotland moved to the area with her husband in 1932 and had two children. Throughout her life she raised her children and helped her husband in the fields. She feels indebted to the area and refuses her son's offer of a home in California.

The friend who cares for her yard is the daughter of a local farmer. Years ago, Mrs. Scotland was one of the neighbors who helped them out and she believes those "good works are coming back to her."

Her family spent little time playing during her childhood. Most of the children worked in the fields. Mrs. Scotland helped her family by being "the seamstress in the hours," and this kept her from spending the same amount of time in the fields as the other children. Much of her sewing was for others, and as recently as 3 years ago she created a wedding gown and 12 bridesmaids' dresses.

As a deaconess, others look up to her and ask her for advice. She does not give advice to everyone because, "You can't tell everybody what you think." As a volunteer in her church, she folds napkins around spoons and forks for church suppers "just like you do in a restaurant." She is a member of the church choir.

Values and Attitudes

Mrs. Scotland's positive attitude about helping and giving to others is contagious to those around her. She summarizes the importance she places on making social contributions by saying, "I feel like I have done my duty when I can help somebody."

Needs

Mrs. Scotland expresses concern that she is no longer able to sew for others.

Goals

Self-Care and Self-Maintenance

Maintain current level of independence in personal care activities by:
- Modifying grooming equipment for joint protection.
- Adding a removable grab bar to the bath tub.
- Providing an exercise video and appropriate instruction for safe use.

Intrinsic Gratification

Increase independence in sewing, fishing, and socializing by:

❦ Arranging for transportation to community center activities.

❦ Adding a handrail to the back stairs for safe access to the yard.

❦ Finding a fishing buddy in the community.

❦ Repairing the sewing machine.

❦ Modifying sewing and quilting action processes to accommodate physical constraints.

Reciprocal Interpersonal Relatedness

Increase opportunities for social interaction by:

❦ Working with Concerned Citizens of Tillery to identify opportunities in the community.

❦ Collaborating with Mrs. Scotland to develop a weekly schedule.

❦ Working with Concerned Citizens of Tillery to arrange for transportation to identified events in the community.

Societal Contribution

Increase opportunities for societal contribution by:

❦ Working with the church to identify events at which Mrs. Scotland can assist.

❦ Working with church members who drive to schedule drivers for events.

❦ Modifying activities to be done at events to ensure energy conservation and joint protection.

❦ Educating Mrs. Scotland on ways to do modified activities.

Intervention

During the limited time that occupational therapy services were provided to Mrs. Scotland, some significant gains were made. Remedial (using the biomechanical frame of reference), compensatory, and educational strategies were all used to meet goals. Due to concerns about her safety, a hand railing was installed on her back steps, making it easier and safer for her to spend time in her back yard, picking peanuts from the field, and hanging wet clothes. The Concerned Citizens of Tillery office was notified of her need for transportation to attend community events and agreed to help with this whenever possible. Energy conservation and joint protection strategies were discussed with Mrs. Scotland to further meet established goals. Ways to have her sewing machine repaired or replaced were also sought.

THE LIFESTYLE PERFORMANCE MODEL AND RESEARCH

Fascinated by the fact that many elderly residents ages 65 to 100 years still live independently in their homes, we, as occupational therapy faculty, decided to study how occupations facilitate or inhibit this capacity. Working within the context of the community, we particularly wanted to know what specific aspects of this African-American culture might be related to elders' ability to maintain their independence. With little available published literature to guide us in the experience and in order to fit the tenets of the Lifestyle Performance Model, an ethnographic methodology for the study seemed most appropriate.

Client Population

Ten individuals have been interviewed thus far using the Lifestyle Performance Profile. They range in age from 50 to 100 years. All but one are female. All are of African-American descent; one is an original resettlement community farmer and others are descendants of the resettlement community. Some have left the Tillery community for a period of years and have chosen to return; others have lived their entire lives in Tillery. All live in their own homes that are surrounded by some green space; one resident still owns several acres of cotton farmland, another picks peanuts from the fields directly behind her house. Economic poverty is commonplace; 80% to 90% of the individuals interviewed to date lives at or below the federal poverty level. Poverty appears to be offset by other qualities in community life. For the occupational therapists involved, it has been a valued and memorable experience to work with Mrs. C., who makes all of her own clothing by hand, without patterns, despite a shoulder injury acquired many years ago while logging her land. Mrs. F. and Mrs. W. tell stories of the cooking and baking they did to raise "20 head of chillen." Mr. G. was an original resettlement farmer who still raises a full garden and proudly serves watermelon to his visitors. Mrs. E. was a persistent teacher, explaining why she wishes to be able to get to church to sing in the "Amen" chorus.

The residents' descriptions of past and present occupations prompted us to further examine the roles and occupations assigned or chosen by the Tillery residents that have allowed them to successfully age "in place." By better understanding these occupations and the roles associated with them, the next generation of individuals with similar background may be provided the opportunity to learn from these role models regarding the roles and occupations that have provided a satisfying lifestyle for their elders.

Common themes regarding the role of occupations in the lifestyles of the 10 interviewees include the following.

Faith in the Lord

An abiding faith in the Lord is a central focus to all interviewee's lives. As a theme, faith represents both a set of beliefs and a set of occupations. Religious symbols are prominent in homes; and praying, attending church, singing gospel songs, and sharing their faith verbally and through their actions with others are common. As one interviewee stated, "I look upon Him and I ask Him if I am doing the right thing and think He answers me." Another commented, "The Lord is with me, brought me back." Another expressed the influence of a higher being in her everyday life when she stated, "I asked the Lord, I said Lordy please let somebody call or somebody stop by."

Independence in Doing

A common theme expressed in many ways by the interviewees is the value they place on maintaining their independence, particularly their ability to do activities on their own. Comments like, "I hate it 'cause I can't do it; I be involved in a whole lot of things. I'm just like that, and seeing it finished. I want it to be done well," represent this value. Other indicators of independence include managing their own finances, cooking and preparing meals, spending time alone, individual dressing style based on personal tastes, and making clothing and home décor such as curtains, quilts, and couch covers. Financial independence and the ability to manage money are also important. One resident stated, "I don't have anybody messing with my money."

Family

A third theme identified by our research is the importance of family. Caring for family is an important role for each of the participants. Many cared for younger siblings and elders during their lives, as well as for their own children and the children of other relatives. Two participants care for loved ones with special needs; the value placed on this was expressed as follows: "People tell us we love keeping her here (at home). Well, if love is keeping her here, she going to stay here a long time." Another commented that "my wife was with me all the way. She worked just as hard as I did." Dependence on family members was common, "so if anything happens to you, you've got somebody to look for you."

Environment

A final theme is the importance that participants place on their environment including natural, social, temporal, and man-made. Participants emphasized the natural environment, having green space around their homes, and gardening. One stated, "I like to be outside; that's where I'd love to be now." The social environment as represented by a strong sense of community was discussed often with comments like, "But see this is my community. I was born and raised here right down the road, so that puts everything into perspective. It's your past as well as your future. So, you gonna do what is best for yourself, your community, your children, and everybody around you." Another resident expressed her viewpoint, "I can't do that (leave) cause I'm indebted to Halifax County, any time you stay in a place 50 years, what can you say?" Additionally, participants often attend community-sponsored social events. Additionally, home environments of residents were expressions of themselves and their culture. Homes were filled with memorabilia, pictures, and religious symbols. Finally, residents spoke of their past, present, and future in regard to the community's ability to endure.

STRENGTHS AND WEAKNESSES OF USING THE LIFESTYLE PERFORMANCE MODEL

Based on our experience in Tillery using the Lifestyle Performance Model, we have identified several strengths and weaknesses when using it in a community-built system. The model provides a holistic view that broadens the focus of occupational therapy beyond self-care. This is particularly important when working with residents who are entrenched in and surrounded by their community. Further, the model emphasizes the relationship between occupation and the environment. The environment is described broadly to include the physical (man-made and natural), temporal, social, economic, and political. These are essential elements of a community environment and must be considered in the provision of occupational therapy services. This was evident in the earlier descriptions of the intervention strategies described in the case of Mrs. Scotland.

The inter-relationship of the environment and person is a shaper of the person's occupational performance and the occupation. This broadens the scope of intervention possibilities to include the individual's strengths and weaknesses and the capacity of the environment to support occupational performance. By gathering data on the environment, the person, and the person's occupational lifestyle, we were able to provide meaningful intervention that fit within the cultural context of the individual.

The model provides a clear lens through which the occupational therapist is able to keep the focus on occupation. This is essential when working on interdisciplinary teams where roles and responsibilities are murky. By articulating that occupational therapy is using the Lifestyle Performance Model, therapists could reduce the territoriality that is common between professionals.

The framework of the model also provides structure for researchable questions. For us, this involves questions about the use of occupation across a lifespan, the contribution of occupation to quality of life, the impact of culture on occupational choices, the construction of a harmonious lifestyle, and the role of the environment in the construction of an occupational lifestyle.

There are weaknesses that we dealt with when using the model. The Lifestyle Performance Profile, a semi-structured interview, was difficult to use—especially for non-skilled, beginning interviewers. The student interviewers found themselves lapsing into changing the profile to a structured instrument, thereby limiting the quality of the replies.

Novice occupational therapists had a difficult time dealing with the all-encompassing worldview upon which the model is based. They were used to a more structured approach using cause and effect strategies. While they subscribed to the value of the broader perspective, it was frequently difficult for them to keep the client's life at the forefront of the intervention process. The research methodology (ethnographic) is time-consuming and requires knowledge and skills not traditionally taught. This required the faculty leading the experience to become both facilitators of occupational therapy services and teachers of research skills.

REFERENCES

Cotton, P. (1993). What can Tillery tell Hillary? Tiny town reforms its own health care [news]. *JAMA, 269*(19), 2485.

Foreman, C. (1934). What hope for the rural Negro? *Journal of Negro Life,* 105.

Jackson, J., Carlson, M., Mandel, D., Zemke, R., & Clark, F. (1998). Occupation in lifestyle redesign: The well elderly study occupational therapy program. *Am J Occup Ther, 52,* 326-336.

20th Anniversary Celebration of the Concerned Citizens of Tillery. (1998). Tillery, NC: Concerned Citizens of Tillery.

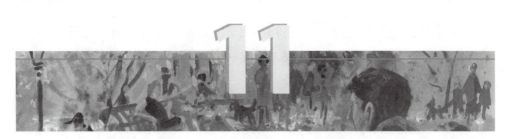

Providing Services to Link Prisoners to the Community

Ernest

Peggy P. Wittman, EdD, OTR/L, FAOTA and Beth P. Velde, PhD, OTR/L

While occupational therapists are well-qualified to assume roles within the criminal justice system, there is currently a paucity of occupational therapists working in forensic settings. Despite this shortage, Cara and MacRae (1998) argue that "the population is compelling and the opportunities are rewarding: the work is fascinating and satisfying" (p. 549). Due to the shortage of occupational therapy programs for prisoners, little published literature is available to guide practitioners who are interested in establishing programs. Jones and McColl (1991) describe an interactional life skills group that they led for offenders. The group was successful in helping participants take on and value more roles than those prisoners who were involved in a conventional psychotherapy group run by the same therapist. Castaneda (1999) discusses the need for helping prisoners with dual diagnoses (mental retardation and mental illness who have been incarcerated) to successfully live in the community and the role for occupational therapists to assist with this goal. Other material that has been written about occupational therapy with prisoners has been primarily published in the British and Canadian occupational therapy literature (Lloyd, 1986, 1995; Lloyd & Guerra, 1988).

USE OF THE LIFESTYLE PERFORMANCE MODEL IN THE MAURY PRISON

In 1998, after reading several articles as part of required reading for a course in the practice of occupational therapy in mental health settings, two occupational therapy students expressed strong interest in establishing and implementing an occupational therapy program for inmates in a local prison. Working with a faculty supervisor, they contacted the local mental health center where the psychologist in charge of forensic care expressed his interest and support for such a program. Consequently, the students were assigned to a social worker supervisor who served as case manager for assigned prisoners in a minimum-security prison. The social worker then served as the on-site supervisor for the program and was present for all evaluation and intervention sessions conducted by the occupational therapy students.

The social worker was initially responsible for finding participants for the pilot occupational therapy program. In order to participate, the prisoners had to meet inclusion criteria. These included inmates who were eligible for parole or discharge from the correctional facility and who did not have a strong tendency for physical violence and assault. Four male prisoners were selected for inclusion. One had a documented history of severe depression; other psychiatric problems were not disclosed to the student therapists due to confidentiality requests. Group participants ranged in ages from 27 to 56 years of age. To diminish bias, the occupational therapy students were not aware of why participants had been incarcerated. Prison stays ranged from 10 to 20 years.

In planning the program, the occupational therapy students and faculty member (hereafter referred to as "the OTs") reviewed the literature for examples of other forensic programs and models of practice that could provide direction. As stated previously, while little published literature is available, what was found emphasized the need for community re-entry skills and a sensitivity to potential mental health issues often present in the forensic population. Additionally, the OTs recognized that working in the prison environment was a unique and challenging part of the program. Thus, because of its emphasis on the environment and its attention to occupational performance in a variety of areas, the Lifestyle Performance Model was chosen as the model of practice for this pilot program.

Individual interviews were done with each participant using the Lifestyle Performance Profile. Additionally, to provide further information about living skills, a Kohlman Evaluation of Living Skills assessment was given to each participant. Results were integrated and used to develop individual intervention plans that were implemented primarily in a small group setting. The occupational therapy groups met for 2 hours per week for 5 weeks; the last week was spent re-evaluating participants and getting feedback from them about the program. Sessions occurred in a small room equipped with a conference table and chairs adjacent to several administrative offices located in the same building. Thus, not only was the social worker supervisor always present, but other personnel were within hearing distance at all times.

Based on the comparison of the results of the Lifestyle Performance Profile for the four participants, the OTs chose to focus on the domains of reciprocal interpersonal relatedness and self-care/self-maintenance. Group activities focused on building skills for listening, problem solving, and conflict management. For example, one session emphasized assertiveness training by reviewing basic concepts of good communication and role-playing participant-centered situations in which assertiveness was a better choice than aggressiveness. Vocational skill acquisition was also emphasized; participants learned appropriate methods for completing a job application and interviewing. In order to address needs identified in these domains, therapists decided to use the cognitive-behavioral and acquisitional frames of reference as a basis for their interventions.

Self-care activities were also addressed. Because budgeting skills were seen as a need by participants, they were given information about the current prices of items they would need to purchase, the use of automatic banking equipment, and the price of contemporary leisure activities such as bowling. The cognitive behavioral frame of reference was used to guide the teaching of these skills.

All participants involved in the program had very positive comments about it, and each expressed a wish that it could be continued for other prisoners. For example, one commented, "The prison system needs this, because when people get out, what are they going to do?" Another stated, "A lot of the things were beneficial and helped me to realize that there had been a great change in the last 10 years." All four participants improved on their standardized assessment of daily living scores and all intervention goals. Ernest's Lifestyle Performance Profile is described below, together with intervention goals established from it to illustrate its use in a prison system.

ERNEST

Ernest is a 28-year-old African-American male who has been incarcerated for the past 10 years. Because he lives in a minimum-security prison, a hot-wire fence surrounds the perimeter with barbed wire on the top. Four guard towers manned 24 hours a day sit on each corner of the 3-acre facility. A maximum-security unit adjoins it across the back. Ernest has free range of the prison buildings and yard because of his history of compliance with rules and regulations. He must, however, comply with a "count-down" every hour to assure that prison personnel know where every prisoner is at that time. He stays in a dorm-like building where he is given a dresser for his personal belongings. While the prison is surrounded by attractive North Carolina countryside, the inside has a minimum of green space; the "yards" are concrete and the buildings themselves are constructed of red brick. Picnic tables occupy some outdoor space and are used often as places to sit, play cards, visit with family members during designated times, and "hang out."

Self-Care and Self-Maintenance

Current Status and Strengths

This domain is more affected than others due to the constraints set by the physical environment. Ernest rises at 6:00 each morning when a bell sounds. Breakfast is served at 6:30; Ernest comments that the food is tolerable for an institution. He reports to his prison-assigned job of working in the prison chapel at 8:00. Lunch is served at noon; Ernest eats and then returns to work from 1:00 to 5:00. Most days he then goes to the gym where he lifts weights before eating dinner at 6:00. Ernest purchases his daily living supplies such as toothpaste, shaving cream, and deodorant from the prison store using wages he has earned. His clothing is prison regulation green or gray pants, shirt, jacket, and shoes; these are provided by the institution. Ernest spends part of his evenings "hanging out" with friends, playing cards with other inmates, and reading his Bible. Health and dental care are provided on a regular basis for all prisoners.

Values and Attitudes

Ernest is a well-groomed individual who, even within the constraints of the prison environment, takes pride in his ability to do basic self-care activities. Prior to the occupational therapy intervention process, he took his ability to participate in this domain for granted.

Needs

Ernest states, "I ain't never lived alone. My mama cooked for me and took care of cleaning my clothes and everything, so I'm gonna have to learn to do that stuff on my own when I get outta here." Particular concerns revolve around learning to budget and handle money, planning and preparing simple meals, and interacting appropriately with others in the community.

Societal Contribution

Current Status and Strengths

Ernest enjoys his job in the chapel, where he says, "I'm able to help other guys come to Christ." While he is actually responsible for working in the chapel library sorting and shelving books, his exposure to those who use it provides him with an opportunity to "witness his faith." He also wants to be a good role model for his brother, who is younger, so "he don't end up here like me."

Values and Attitudes

While the paradox of being a social contributor while in prison is obvious, Ernest appears sincere in his need to be a role model to others. He has kept his job for several years and states that he looks forward to "working on the outside."

Needs

Ernest agrees that he needs to learn the skills required to apply for a job. He is unaware of employment opportunities available in the community, especially those that may have come about in the past 10 years since his incarceration.

Reciprocal Interpersonal Relatedness

Current Status and Strengths

Ernest's relationships with others are based on his professed faith in Christianity. He proclaims that the most important relationship in his life is with Christ. Beyond this, he values friends in prison who are also Christians. His mother has visited him on a regular basis for the past 10 years, and he values his relationship with his younger brother. Though he does not see him often, he writes him regularly. Ernest laughs about his lack of relationships with females and appears uncomfortable and insecure when discussing his real feelings about women. He says he had a girlfriend in high school, but "that was a long time ago."

Values and Attitudes

Ernest values his relationship with God; this appears to be what has given him the strength to endure his long years in prison. He is a personable and likable individual who gets along well with others, including the OTs during the time they worked with him.

Needs

It will be important for Ernest to find community-based support for his strong religious beliefs since these may help him make an effective transition from prison to life on the outside. Mentors and friends who share his beliefs could be a vital part of his future lifestyle.

Intrinsic Gratification

Current Status and Strengths

Ernest's lifestyle, including his occupational choices such as hanging out with other "Christian friends," playing cards that don't require gambling, and his relationships are permeated by his religious ideology. His leisure occupations include attending church, listening to Christian music, and spending time with fellow Christian friends. He enjoys keeping his body in shape by working out in the prison gym and, as stated above, he enjoys his work in the chapel.

Values and Attitudes

Ernest values those leisure pursuits he has developed for himself. He recognizes that when he does not have the structure of the prison environment, he will have to make the effort to find things to do which "keep me out of trouble and I like."

Needs

Ernest is unaware of many recreational opportunities that now exist in a community. It will be important for him to use available resources to meet his needs for Christian fellowship, while possibly finding other occupations that he also enjoys.

Intervention Goals

Self-Care

1. Practice developing a budget for community living; demonstrate awareness of banking procedures, including checking, savings, and electronic.
2. Practice developing simple menus, including making a list of grocery items needed with cost.
3. Using current catalogs, demonstrate the ability to identify the cost of self-care supplies including clothing.

Societal Contribution

1. Demonstrate the ability to correctly complete a job application, including prison history, and to interview for a job.

Reciprocal Interpersonal Relatedness

1. Continue writing to his mother and brother, and share hopes and plans for the future with them.
2. Discuss ways to meet needs for religious affiliation in the community.
3. Demonstrate the ability to use basic assertiveness versus aggressiveness skills in communicating with others.

Intrinsic Gratification

1. Identify several recreational opportunities available in the community.

Intervention and Outcomes

Ernest was actively involved in all occupational therapy programming. While many occupations were done in groups, he was able to identify relevant ideas and apply them to himself. For example, he seemed to thoroughly enjoy the classes on assertiveness training and gave several examples of how he could have used this skill in his past, and how he practiced between group sessions. Additionally, he was given information on recreational activities (such as bowling), in which he could participate in the community. Participation in playing the game of "Life" with his peers helped him identify his values and his occupational choices for the future. All goals were met at the end of the intervention sessions.

BEYOND THE PRISON ENVIRONMENT AND INTO THE COMMUNITY

One year after the intervention program was completed, after reading about the program in Cox and Byrum's unpublished manuscript (1999) and in a school newsletter (Martin, 1999), two different occupational therapy students completed a follow-up study. The purpose of this study was to identify common themes that described support available for the participants in their efforts to maintain a lifestyle in the community. The Lifestyle Performance Profile was again used as a basis for doing interviews with participants since it provided a way of assessing life satisfaction.

Three of the four participants were interviewed for this follow-up study. The fourth prisoner was unable to participate because he did not receive parole. Participants were contacted by telephone for permission to interview them; each was interviewed in their home environment by the two occupational therapy student researchers. Consent forms were used and each person was pleased to be contacted and interviewed. While confidentiality was assured, in actuality, each parolee asked to be identified and have their photos taken with the interviewers. The interviews lasted 1 to 2 hours. Each was tape recorded and transcribed by a third person who was not involved in the study. The results were then separately coded for themes by the researchers. After coding the results separately, the researchers compared results and common themes.

Five themes were identified. These themes include religion, support network, role identification, structured lifestyle, and vocational pursuits.

Each parolee identified *religion* as a very important aspect in his current lifestyle. They all attributed their recent success to the presence of God in their lives. One parolee stated, "I see things entirely different. I realize that before I went to prison, I didn't have Christ in my life and that makes it entirely different. I base my life now on His will and what He instructs me to do." Another parolee commented, "I always think of other people just like I would myself, because I am a church-going fellow. In the Bible, it says treat others like you would yourself. That's the most important thing. It makes a difference."

A *support network* was available to each parolee. Having a support network helped them reintegrate into the community and currently assists them in maintaining their positive lifestyle. However, the type of support network between each parolee varied. Two relied on their family and friends while the other participant relied on his coworkers and parole officer. One parolee stated, "I've got plenty of support. I've got a big family and church friends." Another said, "Having friendships and bonds really does help. It's inner therapy for me, and it helps me to know that there are other people out there with problems."

Each parolee was able to *identify roles* he currently performs and seemed to take tremendous pride in these roles. Being able to identify and maintain roles is a key component in undertaking responsibility. Some of the roles identified among the parolees included: brother, worker, son, friend, parolee, church member, and mentor. The role of mentor significantly impacted the parolees' successful lifestyles. One parolee described being a role model for his younger brother. He hoped that by setting a good example, his younger brother would remain out of trouble and not follow the same path that he did.

A *structured lifestyle* was common among each parolee. Having this type of lifestyle kept each parolee busy and assisted them in keeping their lives on track. Each parolee had a variety of responsibilities throughout his day, including work, community service, and other role obligations. One parolee was under house arrest, making his lifestyle that much more structured. One participant reports to community service at 8 a.m. until 12 p.m., has 1 hour for lunch, reports to work at 1 p.m., and then works until 11 p.m. After this long day, he is expected to be home by 11:30. Another parolee lives and works at the Raleigh Rescue Mission, where each part of his day is dictated by specific tasks and responsibilities.

Each parolee currently holds a job and has goals regarding his future career. Having *vocational pursuits* such as this is very crucial to both the independence and maintenance of a positive lifestyle. In fact, one parolee plans to attend college in the future in hopes to further develop his career. Another parolee works for the family business with hopes of taking it over someday in the future.

CONCLUSION

In conclusion, the Lifestyle Performance Model provided valuable tools for understanding the occupational lifestyles of individuals incarcerated in a minimum-security prison. Unfortunately, the construction of a second Lifestyle Performance Profile was not accomplished. If profiles were used at all phases of the project, the impact of the model's use with prisoners could have been verified. The profiles compiled inside and outside of prison could have provided valuable information about the contribution of activities to quality of life and to avoidance of recidivism.

The prison environment was found to have a great effect, both positive and negative, on all domains. Physical restrictions affected inmates' abilities to function independently in the domain of self-care and self-maintenance since prison-issued clothing was required, toiletries were provided on a limited basis, and medical and dental care were available. However, due to the lack of contact with the "outside world," all participants were interested in learning more about current cost of living and how to budget accordingly. The environment also determined interpersonal relationships, but clearly some choices were available in terms of self-selection of people with whom to spend free time. Limited opportunities for societal contribution existed; some inmates were able to find work in the prison, which met this need. Intrinsic gratification needs were sometimes met by leisure occupations such as reading, exercising in the prison gymnasium, watching TV, and through work experiences. An understanding of the significance of the domains on interviewees guided the development of intervention plans that were successful.

The Lifestyle Performance Model and Profile were also useful as a guiding framework for the follow-up study completed 1 year after finishing the occupational therapy intervention program in the prison. This study indicated that prisoners found the knowledge and skills learned in the group sessions valuable and helpful in their transition to successful community living. It was now easier for the ex-prisoners to participate in choices about self-care, self-maintenance, and interpersonal relationships, such as selecting where to live and with whom, and how to budget income. Support networks were imperative for successful community re-entry; these were linked to other themes such as religion and a need for roles, which helped provide support. A structured lifestyle, including house arrest and community service obligations, was common and seemed to help participants cope with the stress of living independently without the maximum degree of structure provided by the prison environment.

The Lifestyle Performance Model is recommended to help guide practice in a prison environment. As one participant eloquently concluded his interview, "I didn't know anything about checking or savings and balancing or budgeting. As you can see from me sitting here that y'all helped me in getting situated."

REFERENCES

Cara, E., & MacRae, A. (1998). *Psychosocial occupational therapy: A clinical practice.* Boston: Delmar Publishers.

Castaneda, R. (1999). Creating community capacity for persons with dual diagnosis and forensic issues. *Mental Health: Special Interest Section Quarterly, 22*(3), 1-2.

Cox, P., & Byrum, S. (1999). Forensic OT: Pre-release program at Greene Correctional Facility. Unpublished manuscript.

Jones, E. J., & McColl, M. A. (1991). Development and evaluation of an interactional life skills group for offenders. *Occupational Therapy Journal of Research, 11*, 80-93.

Lloyd, C. (1995). Trends in forensic psychiatry. *British Journal of Occupational Therapy, 58*, 209-213.

Lloyd, C. (1986). Vocational evaluation in a forensic psychiatric setting. *Canadian Journal of Occupational Therapy, 53*, 31-35.

Lloyd, C., & Guerra, F. (1988). A vocational rehabilitation programme in forensic psychiatry. *British Journal of Occupational Therapy, 51*, 123-126.

Martin, J. (1999). OT students teach prisoners living skills. *Alliance, East Carolina University School of Allied Health Sciences Newsletter, 9*(1),1,5.

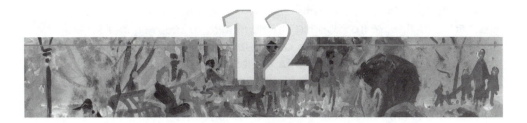

Providing Services for the Terminally Ill

Mr. Pratner and Mr. Smith

Amy Gerney, MS, OTR/L and Beth P. Velde, PhD, OTR/L

Nowhere else in the arena of occupational therapy practice is the Lifestyle Performance Model more readily applicable and easy to use than in hospice. This may be true because the philosophy of the hospice movement is solely focused on an individual's quality of life. The hospice movement recognizes that the quality of life is not measured by the absence of disease or symptomology but rather as enhancing the way individuals spend their time. The Lifestyle Performance Model has at its core a definition of the quality of an individual's life that is certainly congruent with the hospice philosophy. It is this core that makes the use of the Lifestyle Performance Model so compatible with the hospice setting.

Mr. Pratner

For example, consider Mr. Pratner, who was referred to the occupational therapist in the hospice setting of his home. A Lifestyle Performance Profile was compiled with Mr. Pratner and revealed a soft-spoken man who had been widowed for 7 years. He and his wife had entertained weekly, with card games often the center of this entertaining. Since his wife's death, this entertaining has ceased and he has gradually lost his circle of friends, who were "all couples." He fills his leisure time with crafts and became quite adept at needlework. He has two sons who live locally with their families and with whom he remains quite involved. Mr. Pratner has black lung disease from working in the mines. He keeps an immaculate home both inside and out, which he took care of until recently. Mr. Pratner became easily teary-eyed, especially when he talked about his newly acquired dependent role. "Everyone is so nice to me... all the girls who come are wonderful, but I wish I could do it myself." He seemed so indebted to those who were caring for him.

After considering Mr. Pratner's Lifestyle Performance Profile, the occupational therapist focused not on Mr. Pratner's self-care skills, as one might expect in a rehabilitation or extended care setting, but rather on ways in which Mr. Pratner could contribute something back to those to whom he felt indebted. With the limited amount of energy that Mr. Pratner could spare during the course of a day, he made Easter gifts for the staff who cared for him and for some of the other patients of the hospice program—those he considered less fortunate. He gave back something of himself in a way that was meaningful to his need to contribute to the welfare of other individuals and in a way that fit his lifestyle. He was able to accept the assistance from another person and receive the help that he needed for his daily routine because he had something to give in return.

Mr. Pratner soon began giving things away. "Do you know anyone who can use this grocery bag full of yarn?" He went through countless boxes and uncovered a priceless box of memories, photographs that dated back to his teenage years. The occupational therapist guided this activity into a project that Mr. Pratner found gratifying. The occupational therapist supplied two photograph albums, one for each son, and Mr. Pratner began the task of sifting through his lifetime of birthdays, anniversaries, weddings, graduations, vacations, traumas (like the '76 Agnes flood), pets, and just plain and simple good times. Just as methodically as he had once constructed beautiful pieces of needlework, he methodically took each photograph and organized it into one of the two photograph albums, labeling and talking about each one with the occupational therapist and later with the volunteer as he went along. The finished product was absolutely a masterpiece, actually two masterpieces, which he presented to his sons as if to say, "Here is the life I leave behind." He was able to give his sons a wonderful gift.

It seemed evident that Mr. Pratner was satisfied with the memories that he had created and was able to experience a positive life review. Despite all of the limitations that one might have drawn attention to in a hospital setting, the Lifestyle Performance Model allowed the occupational therapist to capitalize on his strengths and create a product that significantly "contributed" to his sons while in the process validating his very existence. This is the sort of life review activity that is so rich with meaning that one could only hope to capture when an individual's lifestyle is truly understood. The skilled occupational therapist is able to guide the selection of such appropriate and meaningful activity, such as this, only when the lifestyle is appreciated.

MR. SMITH

Mr. Smith had a different set of strengths and needs. Although he was recently paralyzed with a tumor on his spine, he maintained an incredible sense of humor and his family never left his side. Since his retirement some 7 years ago, he has been an avid outdoorsman, often found outside fishing, hunting, or just hiking in the woods.

His Lifestyle Performance Profile revealed that he enjoyed many hobbies with regard to the *intrinsic gratification* domain but had not been actively engaged in these since his most recent hospitalization. With regard to the *reciprocal interpersonal relatedness* domain, he was a rather quiet man who enjoyed time spent either alone or with his family. He had been married 42 years and had three sons who lived locally with their families. He had a very closely knit family, and his relationship with each of them was maintained throughout his illness. Mr. Smith has contributed to the well-being of others by taking primary responsibility for all of the yard work and his beautifully manicured lawn. He often helped with the shopping and maintenance of his spacious home. He was quick to help out his children and their families with a last-minute babysitting job with the grandchildren or with a home repair. Since his most recent hospitalization, his son has taken over the care of the home and lawn.

In consideration to the *self-care and self-maintenance* domain, Mr. Smith continued to enjoy eating and fed himself the homemade food that his wife prepared for him. He bathes part of his body, wears hospital gowns because they are easier to manage, and remains in the hospital bed located in his family room where he has full view of his backyard through the patio doors. Although Mr. Smith is unable to complete much of his care, including repositioning himself in bed, he determines when and what he eats, when he gets his bath, and related activities.

After this profile was completed with Mr. Smith and his family, the next step was to set goals. Mr. Smith and his family determined a goal of getting him outside. "If I could only get back outside again," "If we could just get dad to that stream." ("Feeling the sunshine on my face" is a very common request from many individuals in a nursing home or for those individuals confined to their home). After the focus of intervention was refined to the goal of getting Mr. Smith outside, the occupational therapist determined which precursors to performance, or performance components, were necessary to assess in order to enable Mr. Smith to be successful at their goal. This is a critical hallmark of the Lifestyle Performance Model and is in sharp contrast to protocol assessments.

In Mr. Smith's case, the therapist needed to determine how best to facilitate a transfer into a wheelchair, so the therapist assisted him to sit for short periods of time at the edge of the bed. From here he was able to maintain his balance as long as he had the support of his arms, which were strong enough to allow him to "scoot" sideways with support from the therapist. This very brief and specific biomechanical assessment of balance, tolerance, and upper extremity strength was really all the occupational therapist needed to assess in order to conclude that a sliding board transfer was realistic.

The following day, the therapist returned with a sliding board. The use of the board greatly expanded Mr. Smith's world. The intervention consisted of instruction in the use of the sliding board for Mr. Smith and his family, as well as wheelchair mobility. His sons readily learned how to transfer Mr. Smith and how to maneuver the wheelchair in and out of the house and through the yard. The Smiths had a favorite picnic spot next to a loud stream that ran through the property. "Boy, this is great; I thought I'd never see this place again. A lot of memories here." This activity facilitated his life review. This seemingly simple intervention opened up a new and refreshing world for the entire family, which allowed the bedside vigil to move to this rushing stream.

This world quickly expanded when the sliding board was moved to the car and one of his sons took Mr. Smith for a ride around a lake where the two of them once fished. Once again, the richness of this activity could only be shared through a perspective of knowing the individual's lifestyle, from knowing what made this individual happy, what brought him joy, and what was meaningful and relevant in the life of Mr. Smith and his family.

He and his family shared an activity, a simple ride around a lake. It was a beautiful day. They stopped for ice cream. They reminisced. He died a few days later. For the occupational therapist, the involvement was short-lived—it had only extended 2 weeks—but the experience was rich. The therapist received a letter in the mail a week later, in which the son retold the events of the car ride, how he and his dad talked about old times, shared their favorite flavor of ice cream, and expressed the joy that it brought to the two of them.

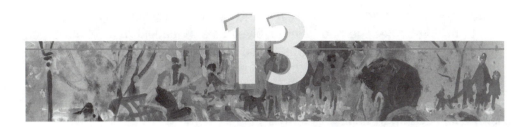

13

Providing Services in Long-Term Care

Rose

Amy Gerney, MS, OTR/L and Beth P. Velde, PhD, OTR/L

The nursing home presents its own set of challenges. For those individuals who have hopes and plans to return to home, the nursing home is but one stop on their road to recovery. It is usually a stop that is filled with a daily routine of therapy designed to build strength, endurance, and activity of daily living skills related to function in their home.

Consider Rose, who is confined to bed with crippling arthritis and who needs pain medication some time before the arduous ordeal of her daily bath and linen change. Unable to "do" much of anything physically, Rose might be deemed "inappropriate" for occupational therapy. However, a close look at her lifestyle reveals a woman with a rich past, a rich history of life experiences typically not considered an important factor in a model focused on the identification of deficits.

Rose is a well-educated, retired schoolteacher who once loved to read. But she states that the "last time I held a book in my hands was quite some time ago." Rose was also well-traveled. She had a host of friends but only a few were local. Their mobility problems prevented much contact, and Rose was not able to use a telephone. Rose was settled into her newly assigned room. Pictures had been placed on her nightstand and a few were on the wall. There were some original works of art on one wall done by her live-in companion's granddaughter.

When an occupational therapist approaches a person at Rose's level of care, it can be assumed that this is not a first introduction to occupational therapy. With

a disease process so advanced, Rose had seen it all—from splints, to built-up uten-
sils, to talking books. She had been involved as an inpatient in a rehabilitation
setting several years ago. Although she had been able to maintain some degree
of functioning within her home, Rose described how her hands slowly "crippled
up" to the point where she couldn't feed herself. "I can't even wipe my nose." Rose
had a full-time caretaker living with her when she was hospitalized for heart problems. The decision to finally come to a nursing home was not an easy one for
Rose, but she knew that staying at home was no longer practical.

Rose and the current occupational therapist had fun constructing her Lifestyle
Performance Profile. In fact, this endeavor was therapeutic for Rose. She took
great joy and delight retelling and sharing her accomplishments and experiences
with others.

When Rose's life experiences are considered within the framework of the four
domains of the Lifestyle Performance Model, the value of this model becomes evident. Honing in on meaningful activities that will enhance the quality of life of an
individual like Rose is helpful to the occupational therapist.

SELF-CARE AND SELF-MAINTENANCE

Rose has not been able to care for her personal needs for quite some time. It
was apparent that the physical prognosis was not encouraging. The skilled nursing facility's traditional occupational therapy goals of increasing self-care skills
were not realistic. This reality is frequently why many occupational therapists may
not consider such an individual as appropriate for occupational therapy intervention. Although Rose was not happy with her condition, the loss of independence
in her self-care skills had been gradual and she had come to accept it. What she
absolutely found unbearable, however, was being, as she claimed, "rudely awak-
ened at 6 a.m.!" Rose experienced it as a disregard for her personal comfort.

RECIPROCAL INTERPERSONAL RELATEDNESS

Rose had a few close friends who lived out of state. They made annual visits
to town to see other folks and always dropped by for long visits with Rose. She
received letters from them occasionally. She had the companionship from her
live-in helper, who visited her when she was in the hospital. Because Rose never
married or had children, she had no close relatives. Her last direct family member,
a brother, died 2 years ago.

SOCIETAL CONTRIBUTION

Rose has been retired from teaching high school English for some 30 years. She
was active in a local garden club where she gave lectures and judged flower

shows, but she said that she hadn't been involved in these described activities for 15 years.

INTRINSIC GRATIFICATION

Rose's love for her students was evident by the sparkle in her eye as she described her teaching experience. Rose took pride in her rose garden. She said that all of the people from her garden club used to stop and see her, but "they really just wanted to see my roses!"

It appeared that there were several components of performance that the therapist needed to know more about before devising an intervention plan. In formulating the intervention plan with Rose, the precursors to performance that were considered were her non-functional grasp, pain, sitting tolerance, and balance.

After some discussion with Rose and other nursing home staff, and review of her medical records, it became clear that Rose was not an individual for whom "improving physical prowess" was a realistic goal. The physical therapist had begun a restorative program for daily range of motion, so the occupational therapist did not even need to make goniometric measurements. The intervention more appropriately focused on compensating for lost mobility and agility and capitalizing on her strengths—her quick wit and sharp mind.

Intervention in the self-care domain included enabling Rose to make her own decision regarding her schedule. Although the meal times were not negotiable, the menu was, so that her breakfast included not hot food that would be unappealing 2 hours later, but cold food—juice and cereal, a breakfast bun, and the like. There was always hot coffee around at 9:00 am, which she chose as her "official" wake-up time; and the juice and milk were kept in the refrigerator until she made the request. Her bathing schedule was changed to the "night shift," which the staff welcomed. Change in routine also enabled her to take her pain medications with food, as recommended. Rose wasn't in total control, but certainly she felt as if she had some say in the decision-making process—she felt as if she was "calling the shots"—just as she had at home for so many years with her live-in companion.

Intervention in the domain regarding *reciprocal interpersonal relatedness* included the assurance that Rose would maintain contact with her friends, both locally and the ones from out of town. Provisions were made to have meals and comfortable chairs in her room for visits from her out-of-town friends. A speaker phone was acquired, and the staff regularly dialed phone numbers for her so that she could talk to them on the phone. A volunteer was recruited to write letters for Rose, with special attention to the holidays when she liked to have cards sent out. The woman who was her live-in companion also assisted with this task when she visited. It was an activity that the two of them shared.

Intervention in the domain regarding *societal contribution* was a capitalization on her teaching talent and expertise with the written word. This expertise was channeled into the planning of a weekly poetry group that was eventually run by the activity staff and incorporated into the facility's routine. She played an instrumental role in the development of this group. Although she didn't put hand to paper and pencil, she generated wonderful ideas, which certainly contributed to the well-being of the other residents.

Intervention in the domain regarding *intrinsic gratification* centered on the poetry group. She derived pleasure from this experience. Rose was also reintroduced to talking books, which she reluctantly agreed to after a staff member promised to make sure that the books were appropriate. Prior to becoming a nursing home resident, Rose had received several books through the mail that she did not like.

The Lifestyle Performance Model is also useful for program planning for entire populations in institutions. For example, in consideration of an entire skilled nursing home comprised solely of the Catholic clergy, the domain of *societal contribution* is a priority of all of these residents, and any facility-wide programming decisions should consider this domain.

The Lifestyle Performance Model is congruent with OBRA (Omnibus Budget Reconciliation Act of 1987). Occupational therapy can enhance individual well-being so much more effectively if an approach such as the Lifestyle Performance Model guides practice. After using the Lifestyle Performance Model, this occupational therapist believes it provides a straightforward approach to achieve the goal of holism.

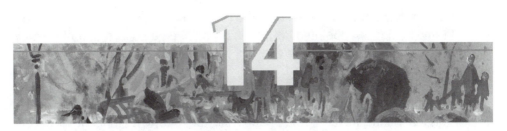

Providing Services in the Community for Those Who Are Mentally Ill

Walter

Gail S. Fidler, OTR, FAOTA

Walter, a 42-year-old single male, was admitted to the mental health unit accompanied by his mother. Over the past several weeks he had become increasingly uncommunicative, sullen, looking dejected, and threatening suicide. Walter's social history describes him as always neatly dressed, tidy, and gentle-mannered. He has been employed for the past 10 years in the local shoe store. He is the only employee of the proprietor, Mr. Evans, who states that Walter has been a very dependable worker, taking great pride in keeping the stock orderly and up-to-date and assisting customers.

Walter graduated from high school, although his grades were consistently marginal. He was described as a slow learner with below-average intelligence, "pleasantly mannered," and with an obvious desire to please. His mother was an elementary school teacher who gave up her teaching position at the time of Walter's birth. Walter's father is a recently retired insurance salesman who had high hopes for his son and is frequently irritated at what he perceives as Walter's lack of ambition and drive. He has never seemed to accept his son's intellectual limitations. He believes that Walter is overindulged, overprotected, and "babied" by his mother. Walter's mother is clearly very devoted to her son, caring for most of his needs and defending him against the criticisms of his father. Such arguments have existed between them with increasing frequency since the father's retirement and, thus, more "at home" time. Walter gives most of his wages to his family for his room, meals, and household maintenance.

Walter expressed grave concern over the problems he causes between his parents. He said he has disappointed his father, hasn't been a good son, and no matter how hard he tries nothing changes. "It's no use. Mr. Evans says I'm okay and not to worry, but I'm not okay."

His parents have lived in the community for most of their lives. This typical small town in Pennsylvania is a mixture of blue-collar workers and middle-class professionals. A small, locally owned paper mill, the nearby regional medical center, schools, K-Mart, and the typical neighborhood stores and service shops comprise the source of income for the residents. Religion is an important part of daily life, and social life centers mostly around church activities and a local lodge. There are two small movie houses, a roller rink at the edge of town, and a recently opened health club adjacent to the medical center. There are several small restaurants serving mostly Italian and home-style cooking, along with McDonald's and a few other short-order eateries.

The occupational therapist contacted Walter, and he agreed to meet with her to talk about what might be done to help him work on some of his concerns. He agreed to several interviews to construct a Lifestyle Performance Profile to form the basis for several interventions regarding Walter's daily living activity patterns.

Because it was reasonably clear from his intake interview and preliminary social history that Walter's employment was a positive, self-competence-assuring experience, the occupational therapist decided to begin the profile building with a dialogue about his employment.

SOCIETAL CONTRIBUTION

When Walter talks about his job, his manner noticeably changes. His voice tone is strong and confident sounding; he smiles and looks pleased and satisfied with himself as an employee. He speaks with pride about his workmanship and his relationship with his employer. At Walter's initiation and with his permission, a call was made to his employer, Mr. Evans, who confirmed Walter's perception of himself as a reliable, competent employee. Mr. Evans has a high regard for Walter's work ethic and says he likes him as a person.

Walter expresses pride in being able to contribute financially to his family and, as he says, "support myself." He boasts a bit about being able to help with odd jobs around the house and mowing the lawn during his father's business absences. He regularly volunteers to help at church functions and clearly values helping others. He stated that he wished his mother would let him help more.

INTRINSIC GRATIFICATION

Walter's first response to the question, "What do you do for fun?" was "Work for Cliff Evans!" When he was asked what other things he did just for himself, that he did simply because he enjoyed doing them, he talked about the occasional outings with his father to baseball games. These are times when "My dad isn't on my back to go to school or get a better job." Walter thoroughly enjoys sports, watches them on television, and particularly values going to the ball park or sports arena for live events. His only active participation has been to bowl occasionally. He enjoys this activity but says he doesn't know anyone with whom to bowl. Furthermore, he says leagues always take the local lanes at the lodge bowling alley. Attending church and its various activities is clearly a satisfying experience for Walter. He watches television most evenings with his parents, but other than sports he expresses no other interests. He says he has a "tin" ear when it comes to music and has never been good with his hands, just "all thumbs."

RECIPROCAL INTERPERSONAL RELATEDNESS

Other than those activities previously noted as comprising *societal contribution* and *intrinsic gratification*, there were no activities that Walter could identify that were done for the purpose of developing or sustaining a relationship. He has many acquaintances but no close friends or personal intimate relationships.

SELF-CARE AND SELF-MAINTENANCE

Being neatly dressed, clean, and well-groomed is very important to Walter. He takes great pride in his ability to care for and maintain himself. He has decided preferences in clothing and derides the "sloppy dress" of young people. His room is as neat and orderly as he keeps Mr. Evans' stock room and store. Since he lives with his parents, his mother prepares the meals and does his laundry and major housekeeping tasks. Gender roles and responsibilities are traditionally defined. Neither Walter nor his father share any household tasks. Clothes shopping, repairs, and cleaning are tasks done by his mother. Walter maintains his own bank account, although this is regularly monitored by his mother. He spends very little, other than the costs related to his self-maintenance.

PERFORMANCE COMPONENTS

There was no need to assess any of the components of performance. It seemed evident throughout this interview and from his medical record that none was a significant deterrent to evolving a personally relevant and satisfying lifestyle activity repertoire.

OCCUPATIONAL THERAPY SUMMARY FINDINGS AND RECOMMENDATIONS

Walter's employment is a very positive factor in his daily life. The relationship between Walter and his employer gives him a sense of competence and personal value. Helping customers, Mr. Evans, and his limited chore activities around the house are significant in terms of his need to help and please others. These activities should be maintained, and one or two additional activities should be explored to further address his needs to be helpful, be viewed as capable, and employable. These might include volunteer activities in the community and church.

Walter's keen interest in sports should be a primary focus in identifying activities within his capabilities and cultural norms that can be expected to generate a sense of pleasure and enjoyment. Opportunities to attend live sports events should be facilitated and encouraged. Helping Walter find and develop one or more relationships around such activities should be a priority. Bowling may bring him in contact with others who share this interest. Bowling is well within Walter's physical and intellectual capacities. It should be a good "match" for Walter since it is culturally relevant, requires only moderate gross motor coordination, and although the game is enhanced through the participation of others, actual performance is not dependent on others. Team strategies and reciprocal behaviors are not part of the sport.

A noteworthy limitation in Walter's lifestyle activities repertoire is his lack of friends, leaving him dependent on his employer and parents for any sustained or rewarding interpersonal relationships. Since he seems to have a firm commitment to his church, he should be encouraged and helped to join the young men's Bible study group. He should be encouraged to join the transitional living group at the medical center. A social worker and an occupational therapist lead this after-care activity. The purpose of the group is to share in reviewing progress toward after-care goals, discuss concerns and achievements, and provide opportunities for socialization and building a supportive social network.

In terms of self-care and self-maintenance, Walter's activity patterns are quite satisfying to himself and significant others. Subsequently, he should be helped to increase those self-maintenance activities that would diminish his dependence on his family, especially his mother. It would seem feasible and wise to eventually work with Walter and his family so he could move into his own living space in the neighborhood. Such a move should be considered when Walter is able to establish those activity patterns discussed in this report.

TREATMENT AND INTERVENTION PLAN

- ❦ Transfer to outpatient status.
- ❦ Reduction in medication with discontinued dosage in 30 days if improvement continues.
- ❦ Occupational therapist to serve as case manager to oversee and monitor implementation of the intervention plan.
- ❦ Therapeutic recreator will negotiate Walter's participation in local community bowling activities.
- ❦ Placement in the transitional living after-care group should be made to provide support and guidance in exploring and engaging in church and community activities and to practice interpersonal engagement skills.
- ❦ Periodic contact with Walter's mother should continue as necessary to sustain the gains that seem to have been achieved as identified by the social worker in meeting with the parents.

FOLLOW-UP

A 6-month follow-up revealed that Walter regularly attends and participates in the transitional living group. He and another member, Steve, seem to be comfortable with one another and have occasionally shared a meal at a local restaurant. However, this is more at Steve's initiation. Walter continues to have difficulty engaging socially.

When his church established a part-time job for a custodian, the group urged Walter to apply. He was very pleased to be selected, and the hours required of him have been adequately managed. This development adds a bit to his income and greatly enhances his sense of helping and being needed.

The Bible study group did not work out for Walter. He never seemed to feel comfortable there and found the reading more than he cold manage. He did, however, hear about and was invited by a member of the study group to participate in a clothing drive. This has led to his helping out in their thrift store.

Walter has earned a slot in the local lodge's middle-level bowling team. The occupational therapist sought the assistance of a therapeutic recreationist in facilitating and connecting Walter with the bowling activities at the local lodge. He is a very good bowler and will go with the team to the regional play-offs. He has gone with several team members to baseball games and has shared a beer with them occasionally. There seems to be a growing sense of friendship in this small group.

The case manager and Walter have talked about looking for his own place to live. He has been reluctant to consider this until quite recently. Soliciting the help of his mother in this endeavor has had a positive effect.

The broadening of Walter's daily activity repertoire and the compatibility of these activities with his personal characteristics, culture, and interests have produced two positive outcomes. Walter's sense of personal satisfaction is clearly evident. He points with pride to his new roles with the church, to his bowling team membership, and to friends. At this time, his mood is decidedly upbeat. A second gain has been the enrichment of Walter's living environment. The environmental settings in which his activities occur are responsive to his needs and interests. He has not talked about suicide or commented about "feeling down" for several months. How he may respond to one of the inevitable glitches or setbacks of everyday life remains to be seen. However, today he has more resources for coping that at any previous time in his life.

REFLECTIVE ANALYSIS

The Lifestyle Performance Model identifies and describes the nature and critical doing elements of an environment that supports and fosters achievement of a satisfying, productive lifestyle. Examining these elements in relation to the interventions that were developed with Walter provide evidence of an enhanced quality of his lifestyle. Adding environments where he can receive positive feedback beyond the job at the shoe store, reducing the time he spends at home and with his father, and the unpressured, natural, interpersonal engagement in the daily activities planned with him has created a total environmental context that is both clarifying of and responsive to Walter's basic human needs, as identified in Chapter 1.

Autonomy

Walter's decision to take advantage of the bowling opportunity, to practice and improve his game, his decision to seek the custodial job at the church, to work at the thrift shop, to discontinue the Bible study program, to consider the possibilities of living independently, and the independence he can exercise in shoe store tasks all contribute to his feeling of autonomy. This is defined as gaining a sense of being more in control than not.

Individuality

The compatibility of Walter's activities with his personal characteristics, skills, interpersonal tolerance, and values has increased positive feedback to him regarding his special contributions. These contributions attributable to Walter include Mr. Evan's continuing commendations about his value as an employee, his high bowling skills and selection as a team member for the regional play-offs, the thrift store asking more of his time because he is so well-organized and dependable, his role as church custodian, and of course his mother's love. This helps Walter to be self-differentiating, to know his own uniqueness.

Affiliation

Walter is clearly a member of the transitional living group. He continues to meet with, get feedback from, and contribute to this group. His bowling team membership and church roles give evidence of an enhanced sense of belonging.

Volition

Walter's cognitive capacities set some limits to his information processing and problem-solving skills. However, within the realm of his abilities he has increasingly used the transition living group setting to assess his options and plan with them. Some of this new learning seems to have carried over into discussions with his case manager and his mother. This illustrates Walter's awareness of his options, his beginning abilities to assess these options, and his use of this assessment to plan.

Consensual Validation

The quality and frequency of feedback from others verifies one's reality and clarifies one's contributions and behaviors. For Walter, this has been significantly enhanced through his employment setting, church activities, bowling, and the transitional living group that critiques and advises him. Walter thrives on this feedback from others and takes great pride in the positive feedback that is directed to him. He is always eager to show off the "results of his labors."

Predictability

Walter does not cope very well with the unknown. Predictability is very important to his comfort and satisfaction. The nature of his job and bowling activities limit ambiguity, and his weekly schedule provides a sense of order and control to his life. They provide for orderliness, neatness, and routine that are so important to him. A clock, a calendar, and a "daily minder" are significant objects in his environment.

Self-Efficacy

To have belief in one's ability to do or learn to do a task provides self-efficacy. Certainly, this aspect of Walter's environment has changed significantly. It is clear that evidence of his ability to productively manage his daily life has more than doubled, extending well beyond his mother and employment at the shoe store. Reduction in the amount of time that Walter now spends at home seems to have reduced the tensions between Walter and his father. His father has less opportunity to engage in criticism but also seems more accepting. He has commended Walter on his bowling scores and even complimented him for his work at the thrift shop. Evidence of Walter's competence emerges from the nature and characteristics of the activities that now comprise Walter's daily living. The performance requirements, the environmental settings, and the purpose or outcome focus of the activities are congruent with Walter's skills, values, and interests. Inherent in such a match is the evidence of self-efficacy.

Adventure

Certainly, the last several months have been filled with new ventures for Walter. He has successfully explored new environments and new social and task challenges, all with a notable degree of success. Again, the fit of these with his values and capacities has limited the risk of failure and increased the probability of his success.

Reflection

Walter shows a capacity for reflecting on and critiquing his experiences. He has adequate time for rest and activity relief but requires an occasional reminder to have some "down time." His need to seek and gain approval tends to pressure him toward more activity, and he needs help in balancing out his daily schedule.

Clearly, capitalizing on and using Walter's strengths, interests, and values has resulted in several positive outcomes. It is noteworthy that focus on these as principle agents for interventions has enriched his daily living experiences, reshaped his attitude, and given him a sense of personal value and worth.

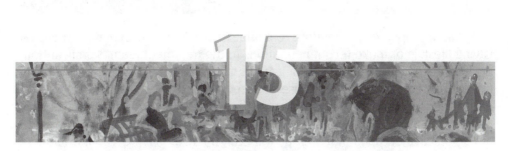

Providing Services in a Psychiatric Partial Hospitalization Unit

Anna

Beth P. Velde, PhD, OTR/L and Mike Amory, MS, OTR/L

The implementation of the Lifestyle Performance Model in the psychiatric and rehabilitation areas of the hospital enables therapists to identify areas of dysfunction in relation to how they impact their patients' lifestyles. As therapists analyze the patients' lifestyles, dysfunction is revealed through the narrative as each person describes what he or she wants and what he or she is expected to do, and how this is impeded by depressive symptomatology, physical dysfunction, and secondary dysfunction. Using the constructs stated in the Lifestyle Performance Model can enable a therapist to view human occupation in a more expanded and significant way. In addition, the Lifestyle Performance Model shifts the focus of assessment and intervention away from pathology and reductionism to holism, a focus so desperately needed in often dehumanizing medical settings. Also, it focuses on "doing" and re-emphasizes the uniqueness of the profession rather than imitating other professions. Furthermore, through using the Lifestyle Performance Model, the occupational therapists increase their overall understanding of how to address important lifestyle issues through purposeful activities. This understanding has enabled the occupational therapists to improve their own practice and teach others in the profession to do the same.

Through a description of activities in the four domains integrated with knowledge about the environment, the occupational therapist is then able to perceive how the individual's lifestyle has been impacted by the disability. The therapist can plan appropriate interventions to enable the individual to achieve a more satisfying lifestyle or make recommendations to the treatment team, significant others, and the patient regarding modifications in lifestyle after discharge. In addition, the intervention plan can make use of purposeful activities that are most meaningful to the individual, therefore maximizing levels of motivation even when the patient is in an acute phase of illness.

For effective occupational therapy to occur, the acute care occupational therapist must become versed in how these four domains of performance play out in the life of the individuals with whom they work and how these domains have been impacted by any impairment. Assessment processes and intervention must account for a person's ability to satisfactorily perform these age-appropriate culturally relevant activities of daily living. This ability is directly related to three main factors: the individual's capacities (precursors of performance), the individual's reactions (secondary dysfunction), and environmental components.

USING THE LIFESTYLE PERFORMANCE INTERVIEW IN AN ACUTE INPATIENT PSYCHIATRIC UNIT AND PARTIAL HOSPITALIZATION PROGRAM

How do those with recurrent major depression (American Psychological Association, 1994) describe their lifestyle? Symptoms of major depression include a depressed mood, inability to experience pleasure, significant weight loss or weight gain, change in sleep patterns, psychomotor agitation or retardation, fatigue, feelings of worthlessness, impaired concentration, and recurrent thoughts of death or suicide. The Lifestyle Performance Model addresses two characteristics that are diagnostic criteria for major depression: a marked reduction in the ability to experience intrinsic gratification and chronic feelings of worthlessness, hence a feeling of decreased self-efficacy. People with depression show a larger difference between their ideas of self-efficacy and their behavioral standards than do people who are not depressed (Sarason & Sarason, 1992). Because of the model's emphasis on intrinsic gratification and self-efficacy, it is important to examine these concepts in a person with recurrent major depression. Bandura (1984) emphasizes that *enactive mastery*, which can be defined as repeated accomplishments in performance, is one of the most significant factors affecting self-efficacy. Through using the Lifestyle Performance Model, the occupational therapist attempts to specifically identify those tasks in which an individual desires to gain mastery. The occupational therapist will then use his or her knowledge of the individual's performance skills to choose activities that he or she feels will enable the person to have a positive mastery experience, thus increasing feelings of self-efficacy. As discussed earlier, the individual with major depression has an impaired sense of self-efficacy; thus, the individual feels incapable of performing many tasks. The Lifestyle Performance Profile enables the occupational therapist to gradually develop or increase self-efficacy in persons with major depression through helping the individual to add mastery-oriented activities to his or her lifestyle. Therefore, using the profile will better allow the occupational therapist to fulfill his or her role with the individual who is depressed.

Another area within our psychiatric program in which the Lifestyle Performance Model has been particularly useful is the acute partial hospitalization program. Admission criteria for the partial unit includes individuals over the age of 18 who have an acute exacerbation of a DSM-IV diagnosis, in which their condition has caused significant enough impairment to potentially cause direct or indirect harm to themselves or others. However, these individuals have enough internal or external resources to keep themselves/others safe; therefore, they do not require in-patient hospitalization or 24-hour professional supervision. Length of stay is typically 3 to 4 weeks, and treatment includes a psychiatric evaluation and medication, medication management by a registered nurse, group psychotherapy, group occupational therapy, group psychoeducation, and individual case management and therapies as needed.

In this setting, occupational therapists are frequently called upon to make recommendations to the treatment team, family/significant others, and patients regarding lifestyle changes and functional status. What follows is an example of an occupational therapy consultation based on the Lifestyle Performance Model in which the patient has many complex psychosocial and physical barriers, which were causing significant depression.

ANNA

Anna was referred for occupational therapy consultation to assess her occupational functioning, as she has been having difficulty adjusting to the many losses and lifestyle changes with which she has recently been faced.

Assessment Instruments

The occupational therapist conducted a Lifestyle Performance Interview in order to complete the Lifestyle Performance Profile. In addition, a physical-motor evaluation was performed in order to assess the extent to which her Parkinsonianism affects her functional performance.

Results

Societal Contribution

Anna highly values helping other people and describes herself as "one who always does for others, took care of the sick." She assists her neighbors, children, and a friend who has lung problems. Typical helpful things she does are cooking and baking for people and visiting the sick.

Anna believes her life contributes to the lives of her sons and their families. She believes her virtues include sobriety, helping others (e.g., she just made food and sweets for a sick friend), caring, and being friendly with her neighbors. She also states that at one time she did a lot for the church. She states that she has a commitment to working on her inner self but that she doesn't know how to do it, only "just being thankful." Some of her life is joyful and these times include when her family and friends are together. Her life was joyful when her two sons were born. She believes that when a person dies, he or she is reborn (she became tearful when discussing this).

Anna has worked a few different assembly line-type jobs over the years. Her last job was at Sure-fit, where she was a packer. She worked until the 1970s. Her favorite jobs entailed those in which she "waited on people," like a cashier job she once had.

Reciprocal Interpersonal Relatedness

Anna's closest confidante was her husband, who passed away over a year ago. She has two sons. One is out of state and one is local. She is very close to her local son. If she were afraid or needed help she would call her neighbor or her son, but she states she really doesn't tell anyone her problems. She describes her dog "Apricot," a poodle, as her best friend.

Past social activities she enjoyed were square dancing, waltz dancing, and big band dancing (like "Sammy-K"). She also enjoyed playing cards for pennies and having lunch with her friends, although she states that this has been difficult because of the pain she gets when she sits too long. She uses public transportation to go to most of her social activities. She met most of her friends through her husband, who worked at Bethlehem Steel.

Currently, she has not enjoyed dancing because she feels like a "third wheel," as all her old friends are still married. She states that she did go dancing once or twice but had a terrible time because she was the only one who was single. This only made her feel lonely and remember the loss of her husband.

Overall, Anna has had an impaired ability to engage in reciprocal relationships since the death of her husband. She has no close confidante since that was her husband's role. Also, she has not been able to build new relationships with others, as all of her present relationships are ones that had been developed in conjunction with her husband.

Self-Care and Self-Maintenance

Anna lives in a townhouse and has lived there for 13 years, since it was built. She states that she is lucky because there is a grocery store and mini-mall nearby. She describes the place she lives as "wonderful" because she loves her neighbors and because it's newer and requires little maintenance.

Her son helps her with the budgeting and money management, and he writes most of the checks. She is independent in dressing, bathing, laundry, and other instrumental activities of daily living. She enjoys grocery shopping and states she is good at this—she makes a list and her son takes her to the store. Although she does much of the home maintenance herself like cleaning, decorating, and yard and garden work, she states that this has become increasingly difficult to keep up with, as she becomes easily tired and needs to take frequent breaks. She generally feels secure and safe in her home since she got her dog.

Intrinsic Gratification

As a child, Anna enjoyed games such as cards and bingo, and she loved to dance (square dancing) every Saturday night. She lived in the suburbs, so she had access to horses and loved to ride. She described fall as enjoyable because they used to butcher pigs and can fruits and vegetables from the garden. She did these activities with her girlfriends. She also enjoyed picking strawberries, apples, and cherries, and then making fruit strudels. In addition, she picked grapes and made wine. She appears to have many fond memories from childhood because she describes an attempt to go back and see the home where she grew up; however, the woman who lived there would not let her in and Anna stated the house looked like it was let go. This was upsetting to her.

As an adult, she continued to dance and met her husband through dancing. She also used to enjoy sewing, crochet, knitting, and needlework. She used to do quite a bit of baking, especially for the holidays. She states that she cannot do any of this anymore secondary to the tremors from Parkinson's disease.

Since her husband passed away, she does not do anything for fun. "The only thing is the dog and when I visit my sons." She also describes sweets such as cakes and candy as something she highly enjoys and eats to make herself feel good. Milk shakes are another one of her favorites.

Recommendations and Intervention Plan

1. Anna demonstrates a decline in her ability to sustain and maintain reciprocal relationships. She needs to meet other single senior citizens and form new relationships. Some suggestions include:

   ❦ Referral to a local senior citizen center.

   ❦ Assisting her in finding out about church activities.

   ❦ Exploring the possibility of volunteering, as she craves being with others and highly values service to others.

   ❦ Atlantic City bus trips: possibly through the senior center.

   ❦ Hosting a card night once every other week, when she can invite "just the girls."

   ❦ Assisting Anna in calling a local bowling alley to find out if there is a seniors bowling league.

2. Anna demonstrates a high degree of unresolved grief and loss, and accompanying spiritual and psychological conflicts. Some activity suggestions to assist her in improving in this area include:

❧ Referring her to a bereavement group.

❧ Encouraging Anna to re-engage in church activities and attendance to assist her in unresolved spiritual conflicts.

3. Anna needs activities that will stimulate a sense of self-efficacy (confidence in her own abilities to perform tasks). Therefore, it is important to address some of her functional limitations. Some suggestions include:

❧ Use of bilateral 1-pound wrist weights to increase fine and gross motor coordination to increase accuracy when doing formerly gratifying tasks, including needlecrafts and cooking/baking. Anna will be trained in the proper use of these wrist weights when doing tasks.

❧ Reintroduce her to needlecrafts such as crochet, knitting, and needle-point, and suggest that she make things for her family.

❧ Instruct Anna in energy conservation techniques to enable her to complete tasks such as gardening, cooking/baking, and card games.

CONCLUSION

The occupational therapist greatly appreciated that the individual knew her intimately. He had a sense of their likes, dislikes, values, hopes, fears, frustrations, and idiosyncrasies in regard to occupations and lifestyle. An occupational therapist believes that human occupation is central to human existence, happiness, and health. Therefore, since the occupational therapist better understood the occupations of this individual, he better understood constructs central to her lifestyle. It is these constructs that enable the occupational therapist to be true to his or her profession's philosophy of using purposeful activities to increase quality of life.

Occupational therapy currently has very few formalized tools with which to decipher complex biopsychosocial information so as to maximize therapy outcomes. It is our belief that using the constructs stated in the Lifestyle Performance Model can enable a therapist to view human occupation in a more expanded and significant way. Doing so would lend credence to our profession's uniqueness within the large spectrum of professions vying for limited funds. Using the Lifestyle Performance Model in these medical settings has refocused the occupational therapists' clinical practice on lifestyle and quality of life.

REFERENCES

American Psychological Association. (1994). *Diagnostic criteria for DSM-IV.* Washington, D.C.: Author.

Bandura, A. (1984). Recycling misconceptions of perceived self-efficacy. *Cognitive Therapy and Research, 8,* 231-255.

Sarason, B., & Sarason, I. (1992). *Abnormal psychology* (p. 263). Englewood Cliffs, NJ: Prentice Hall.

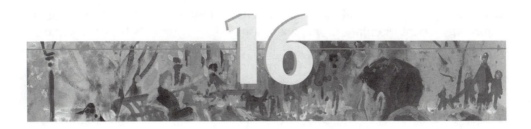

The Model as a Tool for Institutional Planning

Most agencies, institutions, and organizations have come to understand that achievement of their missions is, in no small way, related to the morale and commitment of staff. Attending to the needs, concerns, and interests of employees is consequently acknowledged as sound management practice. The Lifestyle Performance Model offers a paradigm relevant to building such an environmentally responsive organizational entity.

It must be understood that in keeping with the orientation of the model, the singular focus is to maximize the relevance of organizational activities to both the human needs of employees as well as to support the goals of the organization. Neither should pre-empt the other, and experience demonstrates that attention to human needs as an integral part of organizational operations enhances organizational achievement and the quality of its mission. The model views a total environment as comprising the interactive dimensions of the interpersonal, sociological, cultural, physical, and temporal dynamics within which a person lives and acts (Fidler, 1996).

Chapter 5 has described the model's approach to defining and shaping an environment that is responsive to human needs and is therefore most likely to nurture a sense of gratifying productivity. This chapter now attempts to address some of the more significant procedures related to applying those constructs to the organization and operations of an institution. Fidler and Bristow (1992) present a detailed account of the rationale and processes that were involved in changing the management orientation and operations of an institution. The transition of this long-term, custodial care facility into an accredited, active treatment and rehabilitation center was based on many of the constructs of the Lifestyle Performance Model. A summary of the most salient aspects of this project provides a viable example of the applicability of the model in creating institutional and organizational environments that maximize the quality of human endeavor and productivity.

The individuals occupying the 188 beds of this state facility were elderly persons who had spent most of their lives in a psychiatric hospital. Now, relatively free of acute symptoms but requiring daily care and deemed behaviorally unfit for community nursing homes, they had been placed in a segregated facility to be cared for during the remaining years of their lives. Information about the institutions was gathered from on-site observations, a review of various documents such as operating policies and procedures, organization charts, federal and state survey reports, and interviews with a cross-section of staff. The gathered data centered on several environmental components that included communication processes, decision-making, policies of management and supervision, physical aspects, interpersonal relationships, time management, fiscal policies, and external networking. This analysis brought clearly into focus areas of concern that would be necessary if a "user friendly" environment for staff and patients was to become a reality.

Years of mental illness and institutionalization had taken their toll. Attitudes of dependency and helplessness were well-established. Likewise, staff was dependent on management for all decisions. An overall sense of helplessness and futility was prevalent among staff and served to reinforce the passive dependency of patients. Good nursing practice was defined as "doing for" the patient, with self-help expectations viewed as uncaring and cruel. Re-entry into the community was not viewed as a viable option. Expectations for patient functioning was low, and the outside community was viewed as hostile or risky at best by many staff and patients.

An authoritarian model of management was clearly evident. Decisions, problem identification, and resolutions were made at the top and handed down to staff. The physical environment had failed to accommodate to the psychological or physical needs of staff or patients. Furnishings, colors, light, sound, and space were poorly used, drab, and frequently inappropriate. Accommodations for staff especially were limited, out of date, and inadequate. The lack of professional leadership was clearly evident, along with insufficient numbers and interdisciplinary breadth. The clinical leadership vacuum had resulted in limited comprehensive patient services, role ambiguities, power struggles, and lack of professional pride. Low staff morale and the high staff turnover rate were striking. A distrust of management, fear of reprisal, and a high sense of vulnerability were prevalent. Daily schedules and routines, holiday and weekend times, religious observances, and meal routines were, for example, based on staffing issues and budget decisions rather than patient needs.

There were, nevertheless, a number of notable strengths that provided significant bridges to change. The quality of medical and related nursing care was well above average. An assembly line workshop offered meaningful activity to the small number of patients whose values included the work ethic. A viable chaplaincy service, good recreation programs with solid community affiliations, and quality social services with a commitment to family relationships and quality of life advocacy were limited but noteworthy assets. Eliciting the support and collaboration of these few professionals was crucial in planning change and successfully implementing plans.

When these findings are considered from the point of view of the Lifestyle Performance Model, a descriptive profile of the relationships of organizational behaviors and human needs can be developed. With such a profile, it becomes possible to identify specific areas of concern, set priorities for change, and plan relevant interventions. For example, in this setting, autonomy, individuality, self-efficacy, consensual validation, authoritarian management practices, a linear top-down communication process, and the unresponsive and restrictive physical environment regularly threatened adventure and accommodation. The important element of predictability was evident. However, what was clearly predictable was the continual reinforcement of the status quo.

It was decided that if the overall mission to create an active, comprehensive treatment and rehabilitation model was to be realized, the first priority was to build an environment that would nurture and support such a goal. This effort involved "the creation of a clarifying, responsive environment that embodied the very principles that characterize adaptive living (e.g., self-dependence, collaboration, sharing, positive regard for self and others, and purposeful activity" [Fidler & Bristow, 1992, p. 5]). It was acknowledged that only as these efforts were realized could interventions in patient services be initiated with any expectation of success. Therefore, several objectives were undertaken, including:

- Building and strengthening an interdisciplinary staff to provide strong clinical leadership.
- Developing a decentralized horizontal management system, enabling collaborative decision-making and planning at all levels.
- Creating an open communication process that involved information exchange and feedback across the system, from the bottom up and from the top down.
- Providing on-going staff education and development at all levels with a focus on team building.
- Creating an attractive and need-responsive environment for staff and patients.

The "communication loop" that was established included:

- A significantly strengthened and broadened self-run patient council integrally linked to the operation of the institution.

❦ An all-staff community meeting. This forum met monthly with no pre-set agenda, providing opportunity for raising issues and concerns, expressing opinions, clarifying and airing differences, and sharing information. This forum included all staff working in the institution and eventually was self-led.

❦ Therapeutic community meetings held daily on each living unit with all patients and staff. These meetings were the hubs of patient-staff communication for discussing and dealing with issues and concerns related to any aspect of life on the unit.

❦ Interdisciplinary floor (unit) meetings held bimonthly and inclusive of all staff assigned to the unit. Meetings were concerned with all aspects of the coordination and management of patient services.

❦ Bimonthly clinical/medical care committee meetings concerned with the overall directions, management, and coordination of all patient programs and services throughout the institution.

❦ Bimonthly support services committee meetings that monitored the coordination and planning of all non-medical/clinical programs and services in the institution.

The executive committee served as the executive arm of the institution. Membership included all department heads. As the changes were implemented and began to take hold, the second phase of the project was begun. The focus of this endeavor was to build a comprehensive treatment and rehabilitation program that would maximize a patient's potential for carrying out the fundamental roles and activities of daily life in as self-dependent a manner as possible. The philosophy of patient care and treatment relied heavily on the work of Fidler (1982), and Fidler and Fidler (1978). The key constructs of the approach included the thesis that achievement of a way of life that sustained health and was satisfying to self and others derived from the ability to carry out personally relevant roles and activities of daily living. Such activities were categorized as comprising the four domains.

Several principles were formulated to guide program planning and development. Those most relevant to the purpose of this chapter included:

❦ The attitudes, values, and expectations of staff significantly influence the outcomes of intervention.

❦ An interdisciplinary, collaborative approach is essential.

❦ Achievement of the highest level of self-dependent functioning in personally relevant daily living activities is the primary focus of patient services.

❦ A sense of competence, personal integrity, and motivation are enhanced in an environment in which feedback and verification of achievement and contribution are integral elements of clinical, organizational, and institutional behavior.

❦ An environment that exemplifies in daily operations the values of autonomy, open communication, and collaborative decision-making maximizes the potential of staff and patients.

Following these guidelines, the outcome expectations for patient program initiatives included:

❦ Development of a comprehensive, interdisciplinary functional skill assessment instrument.

❦ Assessment of all patients by the unit-based interdisciplinary teams.

❦ Individual treatment and rehabilitation plans developed for all patients based on such assessment.

❦ Creation of functionally homogenous living units based upon patient level of functioning with unit-specific programs.

❦ An education and training program for all clinical and rehabilitation staff focused on program philosophy, program design, and implementation skills.

❦ Development of measurable outcome criteria for all programs and services.

❦ Patient programs that are sufficiently broad to encompass activity repertoires in all four domains of daily living activities.

❦ Improved patient functioning to enable:

   • transfer to a higher-level living unit or discharge to an appropriate community nursing home;

   • or to a community based, supervised living facility such as group home, shared apartment, congregate living;

   • or home and family care.

❦ Full accreditation from the Joint Commission on Accreditation of Healthcare Organizations and the Health Care Financing Administration.

❦ Creation of an acute short-term admission unit to include direct admission from the community.

❦ Collaborative agreements with local nursing homes.

❦ Development of a coalition with state and community agencies to provide after-care programs and services.

Three years after the start of the project, an analysis revealed that the outcome objectives for organizational changes and patient services had been met. Full accreditation expectations had been achieved. The empowering of staff to have a voice in decision-making and planning for change, the authority to manage their responsibilities, the support of strong leadership, open communication and collaboration, and an attractive, facilitative physical environment were among the changes that significantly enhance autonomy, individuality, self-efficacy, consensual validation, adventure, affiliation, volition, and accommodation.

The success of the initiated patient program was attributed to the responsive, clarifying environment, a committed, skillful and well-trained staff, to personally relevant patient programs, and the belief that positive change was indeed possible. Statistics showed that 133 patients were discharged to appropriate community settings in contrast to only 21 discharges during the 3 previous years. Admissions were increased from 78 to 154 with a readmission rate of less than 1%. The average length of stay was reduced from 5.2 years to 1.8 years. In just 1 year, the staff turn-over rate had dropped from 21.57%, the highest in the state system, to the lowest rate of 5.6%. The basic level of living units was reduced to one, with the majority of patients comprising the transitional or intermediate unit levels.

Although this project was carried out in a long-term care facility and with a geropsychiatric population, it should be quite evident that the Lifestyle Performance Model has relevance for institutions, organizations, and agencies. The model offers a protocol for creating environments in which those activities that comprise operations can be maximally responsive to both the needs and interests of persons involved, as well as to the organizational entity as a whole and its mission.

REFERENCES

Fidler, G. S. (1996). Lifestyle performance: From profile to conceptual model. *Am J Occup Ther, 50,* 139-147.

Fidler, G. S. (1982). The lifestyle performance profile: An organizing frame. In B. Hemphill (Ed.), *The evaluative process in psychiatric occupational therapy* (pp. 43-47). Thorofare, NJ: SLACK Incorporated.

Fidler, G. S., & Bristow, R. (1992). *Recapturing competence.* New York: Springer Publishing Co.

Fidler, G. S., & Fidler, J. (1978). Doing and becoming: Purposeful action and self-actualization. *Am J Occup Ther, 32,* 305-310.

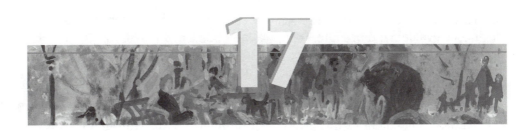

A Look to the Future

The Lifestyle Performance Model has evolved from a lifetime quest to understand and articulate the meaning and role of activities in shaping and reflecting the personal lives of human beings, their society, and culture. The development of the model was the inevitable outcome of this pursuit.

From a beginning awareness, an intrigue regarding the influences of an activity on state of mind–on behavior, from the broad activity experiences in Fidler's youth and her experiences from work with young children and teens in public playgrounds and community centers–came the need to understand and describe the interaction of activities and quality of life.

Activity Analysis, published in 1948 in *The American Journal of Occupational Therapy*, was the result of Fidler's study of 62 chronic psychiatric patients investigating their activity engagement. The differences in their behavioral response to activity versus their behavior on the ward of the hospital led her to question the differences that staff identified regarding their conduct. The activity analysis was an early attempt to offer an organized way of studying the characteristics of an activity in order to understand how or why the demands of the activity were congruent with the needs and abilities of participants.

Fidler's first book was published in 1954 and was an account of patient experiences and an attempt to understand the impact of activity experiences on pathologic thought and behaviors. In 1955, she coined the idea that occupational therapy was a *laboratory for living*. The Activity Laboratory was created in 1966 as a diagnostic evaluative procedure. Hemphill later published it in 1982. The laboratory provides an excellent teaching tool to help people understand their own reactions to and preferences for particular activities.

The book *Perspectives on Therapy*, written by Miller and Walker and published in 1993, provides a good chronology of Fidler's publications that reflect the development and refinement of the Lifestyle Performance Model. Through organized observation and data collection, Fidler demonstrated that the characteristics of an activity significantly influenced behavior. What followed was an ongoing study into how this relationship can be understood, explained, and taught.

While occupational therapy continued to focus on the constructs of work, play, and leisure, Fidler believed it was evident that what was one person's work was another's leisure. Perhaps the constructs were too generalized and stereotyped to understand how they created meaning in terms of daily living.

So then, what is daily living all about? What is important? How do persons describe what life satisfaction is all about? What do the pundits say? It was from asking these questions that the four domains emerged. The first form of the Lifestyle Performance Profile was developed and applied to various populations. In 1989, initial attempts were made to organize and relate the model to the environmental factors using Moore and Anderson's (1968) elements of a responsive environment.

EVOLUTION OF THE MODEL

As Nelson (1997) articulated in his Eleanor Clark Slagle lecture, the Lifestyle Performance Model has continued to evolve as research continues to reform the theory development. The current use of organized grounded theory research at East Carolina University through the Department of Occupational Therapy has resulted in minor changes in the names of the domain, the change in the spelling of the term *lifestyle*, the expansion of the understanding of the environment, and the description of its use across many populations that are vastly different from its primarily psychosocial roots.

Ideas for Research

Where do we go from here? What research would be useful? We need more information regarding the phenomena of congruence. What makes for a "match," a harmony between a person and an activity? Csikszentmihalyi (1990) describes a phenomena called *flow*. Is this the ultimate in congruence? Does it relate to the model? Why does flow occur?

We need research into the interaction between activities, brain structure, and chemistry. Ned Hermann (1988) began looking at this and published *The Creative Brain* in 1988. This leads to the study of "doing." What is this about? What happens in this process regarding physiology, psychology, sensorimotor processes, etc.?

We need more investigation regarding the cultural aspect—how different cultures create different meanings through occupation. For example, is the Lifestyle Performance Model only relevant in the Western world? How would Asian perspectives differ (the model has been presented and taught in Japanese occupational therapy schools)? What of gender orientation? How have lifestyles and the kind of activities in each domain changed during the 20th century? What changes have occurred in the sports taught in schools for women today as compared to the 1920s or 1960s? How do people interpret the value of each domain? Does this vary with age cohorts, gender, and socio-economic status?

Application and investigation into the environmental components of the model are essential. This includes the refinement of an outline or format for assessing the activities of an organization or family in relation to its environment and human need responsiveness. This creates a more user-friendly environment and enhances member and worker satisfaction. Nursing homes are a gold mine for such research. How can this component of the model be applied to enriching neighborhoods, developing citizenship?

Finally, the efficacy of the model must be pursued. When the Lifestyle Performance Model is used to guide the development of a lifestyle profile and intervention plan, what are the outcomes?

Congruence With Social Models of Disability

The practice of occupational therapy using a holistic model with a focus on quality of life is supported by legislation such as the Individuals with Disabilities Education Act (see discussion in Chapter 9) and the Omnibus Budget Reconciliation Act. Both support quality of life as an outcome for persons receiving services through specific systems such as the school and the nursing home.

As occupational therapy moves into the community, the opportunities to offer services to client groups beyond those with health impairments increase. The World Health Organization, through the *International Classification of Functioning, Disability and Health*, emphasizes the important interactions between environment, activity, and participation in society. This social model of disability opens the door to providing community services that enhance the participation levels of all persons. The use of the Lifestyle Performance Model provides the practitioner with a guide to the type of information needed to enhance activity and participation within the environmental context.

The Americans with Disabilities Act of 1990 limits discrimination in the provision of public services and specifies that no qualified individual with a disability shall, "by reason of such disability," be excluded from participation in, or be denied the benefits of, a public entity's services, programs, or activities. With its holistic orientation regarding harmony among the four domains and its focus on the environment, the model is another way for occupational therapy practitioners to uphold the intent of this law.

THE FUTURE OF SCHOLARLY DEBATE REGARDING THE MODEL

While some scholarly debate and reflective analysis regarding the Lifestyle Performance Model has occurred (Hengel, 1997; Hocking & Whiteford, 1997a, 1997b; Velde, Gerney, Trompetter, & Amory, 1997), further investigation, critical review, and dialogue are needed to ensure that the model moves beyond theory into pragmatic reality. Too frequently, criticisms of the model revolve around the time it takes to complete the data-gathering process coupled with constraints of medical systems and reimbursers. It is our belief that continued use of the model and research regarding the model will resolve those objections. Dunn et al. (1999) correctly suggest that, "given the increasing complexity of our work and our patients' lives, our profession must continue to strive to increase the breadth and depth of its knowledge through scholarly debate and the application of critical thought" (p. 400).

REFERENCES

Csikszentmihalyi, M. (1990). *Flow: The psychology of optimal experience.* New York: Harper & Row.

Dunn, E., Schulz, E. K., Schulz, C. H., Honaker, D., & Wiley, A. M. (1999). The issue is—The importance of scholarly debate in occupational therapy. *Am J Occup Ther, 53,* 398-400.

Fidler, G. S. (1948). Psychological evaluation of occupational therapy activities. *Am J Occup Ther, 2,* 248-287.

Fidler G. S., & Fidler J. W. (1954). *Introduction to psychiatric occupational therapy.* New York: Macmillan.

Hemphill, B. (Ed.). (1982). *The evaluative process in psychiatric occupational therapy.* Thorofare, NJ: SLACK Incorporated.

Hengel, J. (1997). Letters to the editor—Criticism of Fidler's model debated. *Am J Occup Ther, 51,* 710.

Hermann, N. (1988). *The creative brain.* Lake Lure, NC: Brain Books, Inc.

Hocking, C., & Whiteford, G. (1997a). The issue is—What are the criteria for development of occupational therapy theory? A response to Fidler's lifestyle performance model. *Am J Occup Ther, 51,* 154-157.

Hocking, C., & Whiteford, G. (1997b). Letters to the editor—Authors' response. *Am J Occup Ther, 51,* 710.

Miller, R., & Walker, K. F. (1993). *Perspectives on theory for the practice of occupational therapy.* Gaithersberg, MD: Aspen.

Moore, O. K., & Anderson, A. R. (1968). *Some principles for the design of clarifying educational environments.* Pittsburgh, PA: University of Pittsburgh Learning Research and Development Center.

Nelson, D. (1997). Eleanor Clark Slagle lecture: Why the profession of occupational therapy will flourish in the 21st century. *Am J Occup Ther, 51,* 11-24.

Velde, B. P., Gerney, A., Trompetter, L., & Amory, M. A. (1997). The issue is—Fidler's lifestyle performance model: Why we disagree with Hocking and Whiteford's critique. *Am J Occup Ther, 51*, 784-787.

World Health Organization. (2001). *International classification of functioning disability and health.* Retrieved 1/2/02, from http://www3.who.int/icf/icftemplate.cfm.

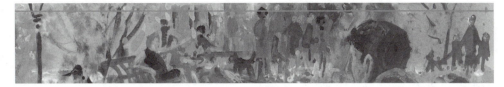

Index

Build Your Library

Along with this title, we publish numerous products on a variety of topics. We are sure that you will find the below titles to be an essential addition to your library. Order your copies today or contact us for a copy of our latest catalog for additional product information.

ACTIVITIES: REALITY AND SYMBOL

Gail Fidler, OTR, FAOTA and Beth Velde, PhD, OTR/L

192 pp., Hard Cover, 1999, ISBN 1-55642-383-7, Order #33837, **$35.00**

This text examines the potential of activities to reflect and shape social, cultural, and personal meanings; to communicate certain physical, affective, and cognitive responses. It will guide the reader to a better understanding of activities and their potential in our lives by examining the processes of investigating and discovering the dynamics of daily activities. Inside you will find an overview of the philosophy and the content focus of the book, symbolic process as giving meaning to the events and activities of daily life, a detailed examination of activities, and a format for analyzing activities.

AN OCCUPATIONAL PERSPECTIVE OF HEALTH

Ann Wilcock, PhD, DipCOT, BAppSCiOT, GradDipPH

272 pp., Hard Cover, 1998, ISBN 1-55642-358-6, Order #33586, **$36.00**

This landmark text examines the relationship between occupation, health, and ill health.

It explores and defines the importance of occupation in life, biologically and socially.

An Occupational Perspective of Health proposes a broad role for the occupational therapist from the perspective of individual wellness and prevention of illness, an occupational perspective of health in contrast to medical or social perspective, and as a major role in public health.

LIFESTYLE PERFORMANCE: A MODEL FOR ENGAGING THE POWER OF OCCUPATION

Beth P. Velde, PHD, OTR/L and Gail S. Fidler, OTR, FAOTA

208 pp., Soft Cover, 2002, ISBN 1-55642-466-3, Order #34663, **$36.00**

Lifestyle Performance: A Model for Engaging the Power of Occupation presents the theoretical base, structural format, and application of the Lifestyle Performance Model. Contents of this outstanding text include the underlying constructs of the model, such as personal efficacy, self-dependency, information processes, examples of application in various settings, and projections for the future.

Contact Us

SLACK Incorporated, Professional Book Division
6900 Grove Road, Thorofare, NJ 08086
1-800-257-8290/1-856-848-1000, Fax: 1-856-853-5991
orders@slackinc.com or www.slackbooks.com

ORDER FORM

QUANTITY	TITLE	ORDER #	PRICE
	Lifestyle Performance	34663	$36.00
	An Occupational Perspective of Health	33586	$36.00
	Activities: Reality and Symbol	33837	$35.00
	Subtotal		$
	Applicable state and local tax will be added to your purchase		$
	Handling		$4.50
	Total		$

Name _____
Address: _____
City: _____ State:_____ Zip: _____
Phone:_____ Fax: _____
Email: _____

- Check enclosed (Payable to SLACK Incorporated)_____
- Charge my: ____ [American Express] [VISA] [MasterCard]

Account #: _____
Exp. date: _____ Signature:_____

NOTE: *Prices are subject to change without notice.*
Shipping charges will apply.
Shipping and handling charges are non-returnable.

CODE: 328